Brooke Shields
Is Not Allowed
to Get Old

ALSO BY BROOKE SHIELDS

There Was a Little Girl

Down Came the Rain

It's the Best Day Ever, Dad!

Welcome to Your World, Baby

Brooke Shields
Is Not Allowed
to Get Old

THOUGHTS ON
AGING AS A WOMAN

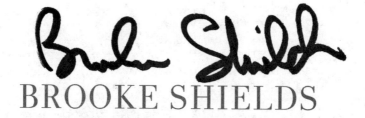

BROOKE SHIELDS

with Rachel Bertsche

FLATIRON
BOOKS
NEW YORK

BROOKE SHIELDS IS NOT ALLOWED TO GET OLD. Copyright © 2024 by Brooke Shields. All rights reserved. Printed in the United States of America. For information, address Flatiron Books, 120 Broadway, New York, NY 10271.

www.flatironbooks.com

Designed by Susan Walsh

Library of Congress Cataloging-in-Publication Data

Names: Shields, Brooke, 1965– author. | Bertsche, Rachel, author.
Title: Brooke Shields is not allowed to get old: thoughts on aging
   as a woman / Brooke Shields with Rachel Bertsche.
Description: First edition. | New York: Flatiron Books, 2025. |
   Includes bibliographical references.
Identifiers: LCCN 2024035132 | ISBN 9781250346940 (hardcover) |
   ISBN 9781250406019 (signed) | ISBN 9781250346964 (ebook)
Subjects: LCSH: Shields, Brooke, 1965– | Actresses—United
   States—Biography. | Middle-aged women—United States—
   Social conditions. | Ageism—United States.
Classification: LCC PN2287.S37195 A3 2025 | DDC
   791.4302/8092 [B]—dc23/eng/20241004
LC record available at https://lccn.loc.gov/2024035132

Our books may be purchased in bulk for promotional, educational, or business use. Please contact your local bookseller or the Macmillan Corporate and Premium Sales Department at 1-800-221-7945, extension 5442, or by email at MacmillanSpecialMarkets@macmillan.com.

First Edition: 2025

10 9 8 7 6 5 4 3 2 1

To all the women in this new era of life: It's an unexpected, scary, emotional, bittersweet time—and yet also refreshingly beautiful and exciting. Please give yourself room for mistakes, successes, and joy. Don't be afraid. Be excited for what's to come. And guess what? No matter what happens, you'll figure it out. You always have!

CONTENTS

Brooke Shields
Is Not Allowed
to Get Old

INTRODUCTION

The first time it hit me that I had reached "a certain age" was while strolling through the streets of downtown New York with my daughters. They are, if I may be so bold, stunning girls. Rowan is a strawberry blonde with curves to die for; Grier is six feet tall, all legs, and towers over me. They're also funny, fiercely intelligent, thoughtful, and kind, though I guess those traits are less obvious to the casual observer.

On this particular day, we were walking side by side, me in the middle, and it was impossible not to notice the admiring looks from various passersby. Over the years I've become used to being recognized on the street, but this time was different: the looks weren't cast in my direction, but at the two beauties by my side. I had every single feeling, all at once. *What are you doing ogling my babies I will cut you but also aren't they gorgeous but also, wait, no one's gazing at me? When did that happen? Am I over?* Protectiveness, pride, melancholy—it all smacked me upside the head in one quintessential New York minute.

There was also the time I was doing a photo shoot, and after a couple shots I took a peek at the monitor. "I think there's some dust on the camera lens," I said to the photographer, pointing to a weird line on my cheek. His response was something to the effect of a pitying "Awww, you're cute." There was no dust. That "something" was a wrinkle.

I didn't have my first child until I was thirty-seven. I went through a hard time after I had Rowan, suffering from postpartum depression, which I wrote about in my first book, *Down Came the Rain*. But with the help of good medical professionals and the right medication, I felt like myself again, more or less, by her first birthday. I had Grier when I was forty, and the ensuing decade felt, in a word, playful. That was a brand-new feeling for me. I remember thinking in my forties, *This isn't old at all! This is fun!* Keep in mind, I'd been treated like an adult (and was expected to behave like one) since I was a kid. At forty, it was as though my biological age finally aligned with the age I'd *felt* for decades. I felt mature yet still playful. I was firing on all cylinders, and at the risk of sounding like Maria von Trapp, the world seemed full of possibilities. I felt like I was being primed for a moment when I could finally pat myself on the back and say "You've earned it!" if I chose to take a break. Plus, I'd arrived at a place of self-acceptance. I actually liked my body and no longer compared it to the runway models. (I never did runway and believed those girls were "skinny," whereas I was considered "athletic"—in my modeling days, a euphemism for "not skinny.") At forty, relieving myself of being compared to others felt like freedom. Mine was a body to be proud of. This body gave me babies! This body could dance! I had curves and was okay with that! It wasn't exactly "I am woman, hear me roar," but I certainly felt like, "I am woman, hear me more."

And yet, as my forties progressed into my fifties, I began to notice that external perceptions didn't seem to match up with my internal sense of self. My industry no longer received me with the same enthusiasm I had come to expect. The vibe from casting agents and producers, but also my fans, was more: you need to stop time . . . and maybe even reverse it. Case in point: at a routine dermatological appointment (to get a mole checked out), the doctor, unsolicited, waved his hand around my face and said, "We could fix all that . . ."

"All what?" I asked.

"You know, all the"—cue more hand waving—"you know."

What the hell? Who asked for your opinion? I thought as I heard myself say, "Thank you, but not yet."

Maybe it took seeing myself through the eyes of other people to fully understand that, in fact, I was entering a new era of life. I mean, I was aware that some things were changing. I get tired now in a way I never did before. I literally can't read the fine print, and I hate it. I used to get mad at my mom for always misplacing her reading glasses, and now it's me saying "Grier, honey, have you seen my readers?" I like doing needlepoint and puzzles, which admittedly feels a bit geriatric. Am I in my mah-jongg era?? I need 2.5s for these granny activities!

And yes, sometimes I put on a pair of pants that once fit, and think, *God, this used to be so much easier.* Or I watch my kids, who can sleep until noon without stirring at the garbage trucks or sirens outside, and think, *Ah, youth. There was a time when I could go to bed without taking a pill or being up for hours in the middle of the night, what was that like?* And though these shockingly beautiful young women spend hours in front of the very mirrors I try to avoid, they still don't realize how fresh and perky and unaffected by gravity their bodies are—just like we didn't at their age. (I mean, the butt and the boobs! How did I not appreciate that when I had it?) They complain that they hate their legs, whereas my *knees* are now practically lower than my calves. How is that even a thing? We are always chasing, never appreciating, and what runs through my mind is, *Ugh, where is the justice?? Why are we forever criticizing ourselves and our bodies while seeking ridiculous perfection? Why do we never see how unique and special we are? And why, when we finally take the pressure off or count our blessings or just enjoy who we are, is it practically too late?*

But while I don't feel as invincible as I did in my youth, I also don't feel fifty-nine. When I was a kid, fifty-nine seemed so OLD, but it sure doesn't feel old to me now! When I say my age out loud, I know it may *sound* old to some people, but I truly don't *feel*, in any way, aged. Aging is a journey full of contradictions, especially in America. It's humbling and surprising and empowering and daunting and liberating. In plenty of cultures, older people are revered. In Korea, the sixtieth and seventieth birthdays are considered major life events, marked by parties and feasts. In Native American communities, elders are often referred to as "wisdom-keepers"—they're considered community leaders. In India, elders have the final word in family disputes. In the Henchy-Shields household, on the other hand, this elder is constantly told, "Mom, you just don't get it!"

In fact, a March 2023 cover story of the American Psychological Association's *Monitor on Psychology* described ageism in America as "one of the last socially acceptable prejudices."[1] Brands trip over themselves to capture the coveted eighteen-to-thirty-four demographic, even though surveys have found it's women over forty who have the most purchasing power: we have accumulated wealth, and we're making 85 percent of the household-buying decisions.[2] The numbers for women over fifty are even more staggering: We control a net worth of $19 trillion, and spend 2.5 times that of the average person.[3] Women in their forties and fifties are treated like we're invisible, even though we're one of the fastest-growing demographics in the country. (One in four Americans is a woman over forty.[4]) We are ignored by brands, and when we are targeted, it's for wrinkle cream or menopause supplements. Talk about shortsighted.

This notion of invisibility is so widespread, so pervasive, that it has become the namesake of a social phenomenon, aptly dubbed "invisible woman syndrome." The gist? When we are no longer deemed sexy or able to contribute to society by birthing and raising young children, our value diminishes. We are overlooked, ignored, or worse, not seen at all.

And the older we get, the more extreme it gets. An analysis of nearly eleven thousand ads featuring over twenty thousand people in 2021 and 2022 found that those featuring women over sixty years old amounted to a whopping 0.93 percent of all advertisements.[5] You read that right: *less than one percent* of all advertisements feature women over sixty, even though the 2020 census found that one in six people in America is over sixty-five.[6]

According to a survey of women over forty by the advertising agency Fancy (which is specifically focused on marketing to a female audience), most women over forty feel that brands "underestimate their spending power and intelligence while overestimating their preoccupation with appearance."[7] We are, it turns out, more than just a demographic obsessed with looking younger. We embody vitality. We are smart and vibrant and powerful and ambitious. We are experienced, confident, capable, and complicated. We are running shit.

The truth is, I still can't quite get over that I'm using words like "aging" and "elder" in the same breath as I talk about myself and my friends. I'm not even sixty! I may not be playing the ingénue or the girl next door or even the first love, but I'm not exactly the grandmother in *Titanic*.

And yet, no one knows what to do with me. After all, Brooke Shields is not allowed to get old. The sixteen-year-old Calvin Klein model? *Time* magazine's face of the '80s? It's sacrilegious! I remember seeing a picture of what Marilyn Monroe would look like if she were still alive today, and it was truly impossible to wrap my head around. But she died looking like Marilyn Monroe. For me, as my body and face change in all the ways they should (don't get me started on my thinning, graying eyebrows), there is this sense of *How dare you? That was never the plan, young lady!* And, to be totally honest, there have been times when it's made me feel like a disappointment. Maybe you've felt this way, too—maybe you were an athlete in your youth, singled out for your form and speed, and now you can still swim or run or play tennis or whatever, but not at the same level. You're still strong, but you had the audacity to grow older, to change, to slow down a bit, to *not* die young or stop aging entirely. You survived, and it should be celebrated, and yet there's a sense that you're not as valuable or exceptional as you once were, and therefore you're letting people down. And these reactions can cause us to feel disappointed in ourselves, too. I look back sometimes and feel like I've done something wrong because I no longer have the body or the face that I used to have. And yet, if I did anything drastic to hold on to my looks from my youth or to stop aging, I'd be judged or chastised for that, too.

Generally speaking, at fifty-nine, I feel more confident than I ever have. I'm more comfortable in my skin and have stopped comparing myself to *this* ideal or worrying about *that* expectation. But I'll admit that even as I'm experiencing this newfound sense of satisfaction, I have to remind myself, sometimes daily, that I am good enough. The old negative tapes are lying in wait in the Walkman (remember those!?), ready for me to press play at any moment. But I also realize that if I don't wear makeup or the "right"-sized jeans and someone has a problem with it, that's on them. And yes, I continue to exercise and take care of my skin, but I think of it now as a privilege, because it makes me feel better. Do I sometimes wish that all my bits had remained higher and perkier? Or that I had the same skin that appeared on the cover of *Life* magazine in 1983? Of course I do! Who doesn't miss the gifts of youth? But this is a body—and soul—that has carried me through *a lot*, and I'm not ashamed to admit that I think

I deserve some credit for this life well lived. We do all this work and get through hard times and suddenly you have a line on your face, and that one little wrinkle carries more weight than decades of accomplishments.

I'll tell you, it took me a long time to have the guts to say that I deserved a bit more respect. Something began to shift in me around age forty. I started to own myself and my narrative in a new way. I'm not sure what it was that finally clicked, though becoming a mother probably had something to do with it. What I do know is that gaining that deeper sense of identity allowed me to speak up when others tried to diminish me. It's allowed me to look within and identify patterns and break cycles. It's allowed me to take on new risks and challenges. I know who I am and what I have to offer, and I've stopped hoping or trying to be different, or something that I'm not.

Of course, as proud as I am of how far I've come . . . there is still so much that I want to do. I want to pile into a camper with my daughters and my husband and take a cross-country road trip (although we'd probably end up killing each other, and the romance of the Porta Potti would surely wear off quickly). I want to learn to play an instrument. I want to get back to being fluent in French (it was my college major, after all). I want to travel to places I haven't been. The list goes on.

All of this is doable, because there's a lot of freedom that comes with age. It's more fun to take a dance class when you can truly let yourself dance like no one is watching. It's more fun to go out with friends when you aren't worrying if you said the wrong thing or if people are talking about you behind your back. It's more fun to go to a restaurant alone when you realize that no one is wondering why you don't have a companion . . . that no one is looking at you at all, because they're all dealing with their own shit. And while, yes, my body is a little creakier than it once was, and it's not as easy to lose weight, the truth is I can still do almost everything I used to do. And the things I can't, well, I don't really want to. I don't want to surf (more on that in chapter 3). I don't want to ski, unless it's somewhere sunny and the trail is long and relatively flat—I just don't feel like exposing myself to freezing temperatures, fighting scary moguls, and navigating with the gear. But I don't feel limited. I'm happy that, at least for me, the moment for more intense, competitive activities has passed, and the moment for new emotional beginnings has arrived. I don't have to prove myself anymore. This is it. This is me! And if there is something I want to change, then I can make the decision to do so.

What I've come to realize—not only from my own lived experience but also from conversations with other women my age—is that these "later" years are all about coming into your own and pivoting in the directions you've always wanted to go. You can finally live the life you intended to, because you no longer have to act in accordance with external timelines, something that is part and parcel of being a woman. I don't have to get married by this date or have kids by this age or get a certain job before that milestone. My time is my own.

And yet—this newfound gift has come as a bit of a surprise. After all, the narrative we've been served for years is that it's all downhill for women after a certain age. As I hit my midfifties, I grew increasingly curious about the disconnect between how this age feels and how it's portrayed in our culture and society. I talked to other women my age who felt the same tension I did— both personally empowered and systemically dismissed. And this idea of being collectively ignored . . . it irked me. I started connecting even more with women over forty, online and on social media, because I wanted to dig into what makes aging hard and what makes it great. What began as an online community to discuss health, aging, sexuality, relationships, and just plain living—to dish about all those things you can't say to anyone except your closest girlfriends—evolved into a hair-care brand, Commence, and a new business. So here I am, a first-time CEO in my fifties, inspired to start a business—and write a book!—all because of society's most uninspiring take on women my age.

My first two memoirs, *Down Came the Rain* and *There Was a Little Girl*, were at their core about overcoming obstacles: first, postpartum depression, and second, losing my mom. But there is nothing to "overcome" about aging. That's the whole point! This time of our lives is something to enjoy and revel in, not something to merely survive. So if those books were about how I persevered through tough moments, this one is about how I took ownership and agency of a moment I'd been *told* would be tough, but really is rich and complex. But come on, life is complex. This book is about embracing an era that has been billed as an obstacle when, in reality, it's a stimulus. Yes, it has new and difficult challenges, but it doesn't have to be viewed as torture or a time to throw in the towel. I'm not trying to stave off this period, or deny it, or pretend I'm not in it. I'm taking the whole mess of it and reminding myself, and hopefully other women, that we have the elements we need to thrive. The story we've been told is, in a word, bullshit. We are the narrators of our next chapters.

For too long, women have talked about aging only in whispers and behind closed doors. Maybe it's because we've been embarrassed or ashamed. Maybe it's because we don't think anyone would want to hear what we have to say. These are understandable responses to our treatment by society, but they only serve to keep us isolated and disempowered. Recently, I had the pleasure of attending an intimate "couch conversation" with Gloria Steinem where she was talking about the challenges of being a woman today. The younger women in the room were eagerly asking her, "But how can we fix it? How can we be a force for change?" And she reminded us that "every important movement started in a room like this—in a basement, or a living room." When we step out from behind those closed doors and use our voices to talk about the misunderstandings, the underestimations, we're already starting to change them. Maybe even fix them.

As far as I can tell, these decades in our lives are a time to be celebrated. Sure, there will be some hot flashes (been there!), but we can wear layers. (Or take hormones, which I have done, but more on that later.) I can tell you that the discomfort of those moments is far outweighed by the delight that comes from making intentional friendships, pursuing new interests, discovering our peak confidence, and giving ourselves permission to make changes to our lives.

In 2023, my dear friend Ali Wentworth produced a documentary, *Pretty Baby*, about my life. Watching it, and seeing just how much I've been through, I couldn't help but feel proud. I'm not saying everyone should make a documentary about their lives, but I hope you can look back at how far you've come, how much life you've lived in order to get to this moment, and give yourself credit for the feat that it is. And then I hope it gives you the jump start you need to figure out how to enjoy this new stage of your life. Because the time is now! If there is something you want to change, now's the time to change it. If there's something you want to stop, now's the time to stop it. If there's something you want to do, now's the time to do it.

Being relegated to the sidelines, as misguided as it is, also offers us more room to fully be ourselves. There's less pressure. We can push boundaries when we're moving through the world without the watchful eyes of, well, everyone. In *Why We Can't Sleep: Women's New Midlife Crisis*, author Ada Calhoun reconsiders all the so-called negatives of getting older. "Could we see . . . our newfound midlife invisibility as a source of power?" she writes. "There are great advantages to being underestimated. Two of the best reporters I know are women in their fifties. They look so friendly and nonthreatening, if you notice them at all. They can lurk in any room without usually wary people remembering to keep their guard up. Then they write devastating whistle-blowing articles. The world ignores middle-aged women at its peril."

At fifty-nine, I'm the one making the calls in my life—not my mother or the media or Hollywood or my family—which is something I've never felt before. And this should be true for all of us. It doesn't matter what you've done, or what you think you've done (good *or* bad), or even what you always wanted to do. This is a new time. The same rules don't apply. Is that disorienting? Maybe, but I like to give it a different spin: We can make our own rules.

1

Previously Owned by Brooke Shields

REWRITING MY OWN SCRIPT

I n early 2023, I got a call from Wayne Gmitter, longtime agent of Broadway legend Tommy Tune, who had a proposition for me: a two-week one-woman show at the Café Carlyle, a New York institution and cabaret lounge that once hosted the likes of Bobby Short, Elaine Stritch, Liza Minnelli, and Eartha Kitt. The regular booker at The Carlyle was on maternity leave, Wayne told me, and he was filling in. Getting me to headline a show was at the top of his agenda. Wayne thought the offer was a no-brainer—a show at The Carlyle carries prestige, and I'd never done it. I'd had a ten-day engagement at Feinstein's, another cabaret club, in 2011, where I performed a compilation of songs from the seven Broadway shows I had done. While the show was well received by audiences, the critics basically said, "She's no vocal powerhouse but she's funny and she's a good storyteller." Obviously that hurt. I'd like to see those critics get up onstage and bust their asses doing something they'd never trained for and still manage to sell out every night! Reading the reviews, I remember thinking, *Seriously, what more do they want from me? I need to be pretty and funny and a good actress, glamorous and the girl next door . . . and now I need to sing like Barbra Streisand, too?* (As you can probably tell, I'm still a bit scarred.) Did I want to subject myself to that kind of pressure and scrutiny all over again? The answer was a no-brainer to me. The answer was obvious: NO.

I declined Wayne's offer. He called back. I said no again. He called back again. I tried to explain to Wayne all the reasons why I couldn't do it. "I don't have a show," I explained. "I'm not just going to get up there and do Broadway standards again."

"Think about it," was his response.

I told my husband, Chris, that Wayne had called with an offer, and I shared my reservations. His immediate reaction? "You have to do it. It's The Carlyle!"

"You're supposed to tell me that I don't have to do anything I don't want to," I responded.

"You'll be great," he said. He brushed it off as such an easy undertaking.

Then Tommy Tune called. Tommy is a longtime mentor of mine. He cast me in *Grease*, where I played Rizzo, in one of the earliest examples of Broadway stunt casting. (I felt guilty about it at first, because I knew I was taking a job from real triple-threat actors, but I also knew my purpose and countered any judgment about my casting by working my ass off. I may not have been the most seasoned Broadway performer in the room, but I could study and learn from the best while keeping a show from closing by filling the seats and doing all the press. No one could beat me when it came to work ethic.) Tommy is the reason why I have a Broadway history and career, so when he talks, I listen. "Brooke, you can't say no," he said. "I believe in you."

There were, as far as I could tell, a million reasons to say no. First of all, it costs the headliner money. You pay for the band, the orchestrations, the writing, the director. Also, I didn't need it. It wasn't like I was trying to rebrand my career as a cabaret star. It wasn't necessarily on my bucket list, and honestly I worried people would judge me harshly once again. But at the end of the day, every excuse I came up with was pretty lame. It wasn't like my schedule didn't allow for a two-week engagement. (As it happened, the show's run took place during the SAG-AFTRA strike, so I was lucky to be working at all. Theater is a different guild, which meant I wasn't violating any union guidelines.) It didn't take place out of town. I lived a twenty-minute Uber ride away from The Carlyle, maybe thirty minutes in today's traffic. If singing was something I hated doing or didn't get enjoyment from, even then it would seem more reasonable to say no, but the truth is that I love to sing! And when I sing songs that are in my range, I'm really proud of my sound. Plus, the skills that come from doing a one-woman show are something I wanted in my toolbox as a performer.

No, none of these were reasons not to do the show. There was a much simpler, and much deeper, reason why I was resisting: I was scared. I knew, deep down, that I was afraid of being critiqued; afraid of not finding my unique sound, one that was independent of the Broadway characters I had played in the past. Afraid of facing my own insecurities. Afraid, ultimately, of failing.

Before I go any further, let me be clear that this is not a "say yes to everything" book. One of the joys of getting older, as far as I can tell, is the ability to say no to the things you don't want to do. It's empowering to know what you want and go after it, but it's just as empowering and important to know what you *don't* want. It has taken me a loooooong time, and plenty of therapy, to understand that I don't have to take every opportunity that comes my way just to keep proving my talent. I know, finally, that declining an offer doesn't mean that I'm giving up, or that I'm a failure, or that I'm not ambitious. I used to think sleeping in was lazy—it meant that you weren't maximizing your day. You could have used that time to exercise or clean your closet! Today I say, fuck that—sleep in! Enjoy it. But saying no to something I *do* want to do, out of fear alone? That ate away at me. It seemed senseless. It wasn't how I'd lived my life thus far. In fact, that's long been an MO of mine: if something scares you it probably means you should do it, because you'll feel so good about it afterward.

Ultimately, I realized, I was terrified enough that I had to say yes. Well, shit.

Doing a one-woman show at this point in my life felt almost symbolic. In many ways, independence was the one thing I had been missing for the bulk of my existence. So much of my life had been lived in relation to other people. My mother, my husband, my kids. My mom was a hugely controlling force in my life. I used to think that if she died, I would die. That was how tethered I felt to her. When I married my first husband, Andre Agassi, I walked into another controlling, rigid relationship, and for a while I did whatever he said. Divorcing him, and then losing my mother, put me on a journey of investigating what I guess is life's big question: Who am I? But in the time between the divorce and my mother's death, I'd gotten married, again, and had kids—so the answer seemed to be "I'm Rowan and Grier's mom. Chris's wife."

And then Rowan went to college, and Grier became a teenager who was perfectly capable of fending for herself, and I woke up one morning and felt hit over the head with the notion that *Oh God, I have no context for this period of my life.* When I was a kid, I was always expected to act older—be more mature, more sophisticated, handle the situation, deal with his or her addiction, be the professional. And it was so important to me, back then, to prove I could do it. All of it. I could achieve achieve achieve in my career and outside of it. I was an old soul in a young kid's body, in part because I had to be but also because it seemed to be my nature. I couldn't be derailed! (Rowan has this, too. She came out of the womb like a shark. The first thing she did upon entering the world was case the joint. I remember my girlfriend Lyda, who was in the room when both my daughters were born, saying, "Oh my god, she looks so unimpressed.")

When I finally had kids of my own and got to sit on the floor and play with them, it all felt so new and joyous; my life felt full. But my kids no longer need me in the same way. When I go to their school, I see the younger moms meeting for coffee and having play-dates, a reminder that, *oh, I'm not at that stage of life anymore.* My husband is a wonderful partner and we've always been support-ive of each other's independence—but my role as a wife has also evolved, now that we aren't raising children together so much as witnessing their young adulthood together (though luckily he's never expected me to cook a family dinner every night, as I don't have that gene, so there's no change there). It's freeing not to have external pressures or timelines around marriage or fertility or parenting, but it's also confusing. I think it's human nature to try to understand your place in the order of things, and my place felt increasingly unclear. It felt like this . . . limbo, maybe. Or nirvana. Or hell?!? I couldn't tell, or I couldn't decide. I'm not trying to wax philosophical, but as I entered my midfifties, I very much wondered, or at least felt like the world was wonder-ing: if I no longer have working, producing ovaries, and if I'm not saying yes to society or someone else's desires or needs, do I have value? If the same familiar rules don't exist for this period of my life, do *I* exist?

Finding yourself in that nebulous place, in that wondering, is uncomfortable because it's unfamiliar. For years, I'd just put my head down and moved forward, checking off the boxes on the timeline of how it's expected a woman should live her life. Yes,

I know mine hasn't exactly been typical—I had my first job a month before I turned one, I starred in my first movie at nine—but I've held myself to the same standards as many of my peers. I went to college, went back to work, got married, had kids, raised them. And I'm still moving forward, but something major has shifted. I used to put everybody else's needs ahead of my own. As a kid I was constantly burdened by obligations, whether to family, societal pressure, the demands of my industry, or even the public's expectations of who I was supposed to be. Then children entered the picture and—poof!—I practically became a robot. I may not have cooked all the meals or driven the car-pools or attended every sporting event, but I was still the one the kids wanted and needed whenever anything went wrong . . . or right. I was MOM. I was the comforter, the fixer, the healer, the listener, the juggler of all things family. And now, for the first time in over fifty years, I have become the hub of the wheel for myself rather than only what keeps everyone else's lives spinning. And this new normal is, at least initially, as scary as it is liberating. Motherhood is an identity, but it's also a shield. I can't tell you how many times I've hidden behind the fact that I'm a mom. Who among us hasn't used "I can't because of the kids" to get out of social plans, or "I'm just going to put the baby down" as an exit strategy to get out of a room full of company that you just can't handle anymore? (And then you curl up in bed and pass out next to your delicious baby.) Children can be the best excuse in the world.

Finding yourself in a period where you are no longer needed in the same ways may not only free you up to focus on other activities and yourself but it also forces you to confront yourself. To own up to who you are, and what you want or need. Now, if I want to leave a dinner party, I have to say "You know what, excuse me, I've got a big day tomorrow and I need to get my rest." It's like

I'm parenting myself—constantly checking in and asking, *What do I like about this? What do I not like? What do I want to do just for me?* It's gratifying and empowering, but it's also awkward sometimes, the idea of putting my needs first and articulating them to others. It's a skill I'm working on.

Given this new reality of my entire existence evolving into a one-woman enterprise, it seemed fitting to find myself thinking through a one-woman show for the cabaret stage. So, I called Wayne. Again. And I said yes. "But," I cautioned, "I'm saying yes on the condition that I can find my own sound. I don't want to sing the same old standards. I want to sing the songs I love and am good at vocally and that resonate with me. I want to tell my own stories." And here the second blatant metaphor was not lost on me, as the autonomy of middle age requires finding your own voice. This was an incredible, albeit very public and high-stakes, opportunity to do just that. Carlyle, here I come.

My stories started with the tale of a maroon two-door 1983 Mercedes SEC. My first car. I bought it with my own money, two years after starring in *Endless Love*, and I used that car to drive back and forth from New York to New Jersey, where I went to high school. Fast-forward about thirty years, when a woman at a Starbucks recognized me and asked if she could show me a photo. I thought she was about to whip out a picture of herself dressed as me for Halloween (it wouldn't have been the first time). Instead, she showed me a photo she took of a maroon 1983 Mercedes SEC she'd seen in New Jersey the day before. It had a FOR SALE sign in the back window, and at the bottom of the sign were the words: PREVIOUSLY OWNED BY BROOKE SHIELDS.

The seller wasn't lying. I recognized the car immediately. It still had the I ❤ GSTAAD bumper sticker I'd put on it as a teenager. My mother and I had gone with Dodi Fayed (God rest his beautiful soul) on a ski trip in Gstaad, Switzerland, and I got the sticker in a local shop. I felt so international and a part of the jet set with that sticker. It didn't quite translate next to the many Springsteen-stickered Trans Ams in the Dwight Englewood high school parking lot, but I was proud anyway.

The car in the photo was totally my car. My mom had sold it to a guy in Jersey City after I graduated college and was living more permanently in Manhattan.

"Pfft, 'previously owned by Brooke Shields'? Like that's going to make the car run any better," the woman felt the need to add. She did have a point, but in our fame-obsessed world, I guess the owner hoped the car's provenance would help it fetch a better price. It got me thinking of all the other parts of my life that had been either sold off or given away over the years. So I bought the car back! I decided to use it, and that sign, as inspiration for the title of my Carlyle show.

For decades, much of my life had been owned by other people. My mother. The media. Hollywood. Fans. My husbands. My kids. Loss. The show, in many respects, was about thoroughly getting back on my feet and reclaiming my life. If I wasn't previously owned by Brooke Shields, I certainly am now.

So much of my identity was wrapped up in my career that the last decade has at times felt like a slap in the face. Agents often tell me that I am "of a certain age" and no longer the love interest. (No shit. But news flash, I don't wish to be.) I mostly get seen for parts that are mothers of kids older than my own. But my gripe with these roles is rarely the age of the characters so much as that the parts have no meat. No substance. I'll read them thinking, *Wait a minute, I'm so much more interesting now than I was back when I was being offered the ingenue roles. Why are these parts so one-dimensional?* But in the eyes of Hollywood I am in no-man's-land. As an actress in your forties or fifties, you aren't Bridget Jones but you aren't Miss Daisy, and so you languish. The stories for women in midlife are about wives who've been cheated on because, yes, they're getting old, or sometimes you get the bitchy boss-type part—the older, insecure woman who bullies the heroine. Where can we watch depictions of the complex, layered lives that women actually live? Where are the on-screen narratives for women in their prime?

Before you write me off for wallowing in self-pity, let me point out that it's not just in my head, and I am not alone. A 2019 study conducted in partnership with the Geena Davis Institute on Gender in Media and the first global study of its kind examined representations of "older adults" in 2019's top-grossing films in the United States, Germany, France, and the UK. First of all, the title of the report on the study's findings should tell you all you need to know: "Frail, Frumpy, and Forgotten: A Report on the Movie Roles of Women of Age."[1] What the actual fuck?

The report found that women over fifty were cast in exactly zero percent of movie leads that year. Of the movie characters over fifty (which made up 20 percent of all characters), only 25 percent were women. Translation: only 5 percent of characters on-screen were women over fifty. And these characters were disproportionately depicted as "senile," "homebound," "feeble," and "frumpy." It's a truly absurd portrayal, and so far from today's reality. Consider that by 2030, older adults (in this case, over fifty) are expected to outnumber children under ten. The 2022 US life expectancy for women was 80.2,[2] which means fifty-year-olds have a good three decades to go, and forty-year-olds are only just hitting the midpoint. A bit of a long time to take to the bed, no?

Another study of women on-screen, this one of women in

TV, had similar findings. According to this study,[3] 42 percent of major female characters on a broadcast show were women in their thirties, while women in their forties made up only 15 percent of that group, and women in their fifties only 8 percent. (Streaming was basically the same, going from 33 percent for the thirtysomethings to 14 percent for forties.) Entertainment is only one medium, but it both represents and influences how we perceive women of a certain age. Still, let's look at other industries. Surveys find that women over forty feel ignored by the fashion industry and the beauty industry—clothes are for teenagers looking for crop tops or they're "old lady frocks" that are completely out of touch with what anyone I know wants to wear. On the beauty side, let's just say that my money is good for more than just anti-aging serum. I'm not trying to look like my daughter, but I do want to look my best, and I know I'm not alone in that. In general, it's been estimated that less than 5 percent of advertising dollars are targeted to adults aged thirty-five to sixty-four,[4] which is obviously the group who can actually spend. How many eighteen-to-thirty-four-year-olds do you know with substantial disposable income?

The problem is bigger than just media and marketing representation. Most significantly, researchers say that global datasets, which inform social, economic, and environmental policies of governments, NGOs, and UN agencies, often include only women through age forty-nine, or those "of reproductive age."[5] A story in the *New York Times* about what we do, and still do not, know about menopause pointed out a survey sent to medical residents found that "20 percent of them had not heard a single lecture on the subject of menopause."[6] Other research finds that only one in five OB-GYN residents have had any menopause training[7] . . . even though half the population will experience it at some point.

This research infuriates me—and I hope it infuriates other

women, at least enough to force some change. My experience of midlife has been completely out of sync with any of it. I felt all the "where do I belong" confusion that one might expect in a society that tells us we have no place, but when I tuned out the noise and looked only inside, I knew I felt stronger than ever. Funnier than ever. Wiser and braver and sillier and more fun and more confident. Of all the research I've seen on women over forty here's what resonates with me, from a *Monitor on Psychology* cover story titled "The Mind at Midlife": "The adult brain seems to be capable of rewiring itself well into middle age, incorporating decades of experiences and behaviors. Research suggests, for example, the middle-aged mind is calmer, less neurotic, and better able to sort through social situations. Some middle-agers even have improved cognitive abilities."[8] Yes! That sounds more like me.

It's easy, maybe even fun, to perpetuate the narrative of the fortysomething or fiftysomething woman in full-blown midlife crisis. *Look at that lady, she's sweating through her clothes and she can't use technology!* It's a lazy storyline but good for a laugh. I get it. Har har. But here's what I think is really happening: this is a story that was written by men. Research shows that happiness in adults generally follows a U shape. You start happy, you end happy, and somewhere in the middle things take a big dip. But that dip, for women, comes at age forty. From there, things start looking up! This era of forty-plus really is when things get easier, or maybe it's just that we feel better equipped, but either way, happiness is on the upswing. For men, research shows, the bottom of the U comes at age fifty.[9] Could it be that the narrative we've been fed of the irrelevant fifty-year-old woman is really just a product of men feeling their worst at this time? Might it be that they just assumed we're bummed out, too, but never took the time to ask?

Putting on a two-week one-woman show was not going to right the course of decades of misrepresentation and misguided data collection or poorly directed advertising dollars. It was not going to force casting agents or screenwriters to rethink parts for women over forty, or even parts for this particular woman over forty, and that was never its intention. It did, however, force me to think about who I am now and who I want to present to the world. If the *Pretty Baby* documentary allowed me to look back at who I was with more clarity, then my show *Previously Owned by Brooke Shields* encouraged me to look at who I am now.

So, who am I now? To start, I am ambitious. I want to do good and interesting work. I once thought ambition was a bad thing, that it meant I was greedy. I thought that there was an allotment of good things, and once you had too much, something else would get taken away. I was afraid to want more because of those checks and balances. But now I'm happy to admit that I want more in my life and am not inclined to settle for less. I want to keep adding skills to my arsenal. And as ambitious as I am about work, I am just as ambitious about leisure. I used to think leisure was idleness, but now I believe wholeheartedly in the value of doing something "just" because you enjoy it.

I am inquisitive. I'm not afraid to admit when I don't know something. I used to think I had to know everything, that I had to prove I could do it all on my own. I needed everyone to know that I had brains, because I wanted to stick it to everyone who assumed I was just a pretty face. But starting my business has only reinforced that there's so much I don't know, and I find it so exciting.

I am a dedicated worker. I like hard work and the reward of it. I like the feeling of achieving what I set out to do.

I am funny. I used to wave off the effort or skill that comedy requires because drama, in my business, is considered the higher art form, but now I can appreciate that it's really freaking hard to be funny, and I'm quite good at it.

I'm a good friend.

I'm a good mom.

I am talented.

I'm getting better at admitting these things that I'm good at, I can appreciate myself, and that's a skill in itself. I used to think it was vain. Back when I was in high school and college, if I got anything less than an A I would leave it out for all to see and broadcast all the ways I screwed up, but then if I got an A, I would hide it away in my desk. I wouldn't celebrate it or draw any attention to my success. Why did I punish myself like that? To what end? I think as young women, we are often sent the message that in order to be successful, we must be modest, we must be humble, we must keep ourselves small. That approach, for me, started early and became ingrained—I'm still working on unlearning it. I'm curious as to when these attitudes start and who, besides us, perpetuates them.

Previously Owned by Brooke Shields opened at The Carlyle on September 12, 2023. I wore an apricot satin dress with a giant bow by Isaac Mizrahi, who sat in the audience alongside Alan Cumming, Laura Dern, Mariska Hargitay, Naomi Watts, and Billy Crudup. My husband heckled me from the audience (I loved it!), and Grier attended in a Badgley Mischka dress that I'd worn in 2001 to an event at the Chicago Theatre. It was, literally, previously owned by Brooke Shields.

I found I had many stories to tell. I performed ten numbers, including Bob Dylan's "Most of the Time" and Tina Dico's "Count to Ten" in between stories about my mother and my kids and my experiences with the likes of George Michael and Michael Jackson and Donald Trump. Some of my particularly odd moments made it into an original song, with music and lyrics written by Amanda

Green and Matt Sklar. The song was fittingly called "Fame Is Weird."

I worked so hard on that show. *So hard.* I logged hours upon hours with the director and the writer and musical director and my vocal coach, who would often remind me of the importance of being "tubular." Our vocal tract is a tube that extends from the larynx to the lips, she said. In singing, being tubular basically means sending the sound upward in a way that it will travel through the tube cleanly. It's like playing Operation, where you have to extract the wishbone or the spare ribs without hitting the sides. When you are totally tubular, you are as centered as you can possibly be, and thus you are your strongest. Talk about a metaphor. I have felt like a pinball for my entire life, bouncing and adapting and trying to preempt bad outcomes and always being on guard, but now I feel more tubular and balanced, so that even if someone tried to knock me over, I'd just pop back up.

There were certainly times when that show tried to knock me over. I ran myself ragged in the lead-up to opening night and got sick enough to land myself in the hospital a few days before the debut, which forced me to cancel two out-of-town rehearsal shows in Indianapolis (more on that in a bit). But I was always taught that the show must go on! So I did opening night with bronchitis.

I wanted the show to be perfect. I wanted to prove to myself that I could do this thing that terrified me, and I wanted to prove myself to others, too. I'd be lying if I said a part of me didn't care to remind the world of my versatility as an artist. But then I worked myself up so much in that pressure to be perfect that I started comparing myself to people who do cabaret work for a living, and that was a real emotional battle. Eventually I had to shift the goal from perfection to enjoyment, and admittedly that one was often hard to achieve. But I kept trying, and when a negative thought wafted into my psyche, I would physically shake my head no and redirect my focus to the lyrics of the song.

In the fictionalized, picture-perfect story of this one-woman show—the nice little story wrapped up in a bow—I would have decided to face my fear, and I would have worked really hard and knocked it out of the park and finished with a proud smile and a sense that I had conquered the world. I'd want to do one-woman shows forever! But that would be a dishonest, or at least a heavily filtered, version of what happened. Real life is not like that. Just because you decide to conquer a fear doesn't mean you will immediately feel empowered. You can say "OK, I'm going to own it!" But if you've been playing the tapes in your head for decades—that you're not good enough, or don't deserve this, or need to prove yourself to those who doubt you—they don't immediately go quiet. The stories you've been telling yourself for a lifetime have a way of sticking around.

By the end of my run at The Carlyle, many wonderful things had happened. It was a completely sold-out run, I was asked to return to do another show, and there was a review that called the show "a true musical spectacular" and went on to say that I had "both a good sense of humor and quite a nice voice." (I'll happily take that and replace the old review that was etched in my mind.) And yet, my feeling when it was over wasn't *Wow, I love this and can't wait to do this again!* It was more like, *Well, I don't dread this, but do I thrive in this environment? Do I really love it?* I'm so proud of myself for not letting the fear of failing stop me. I mean come on, Brooke, you just did a one-woman show and you didn't sob afterward! Even when I felt like my voice wasn't its strongest, I didn't beat myself up. I accepted that I don't have to be perfect to do a good job. And that kind of acceptance—not resignation, but true acceptance—feels like an accomplishment of its own.

The story where "I did the scary thing and it turns out I love it!" and then the credits roll is, in my opinion, far less interesting than what really happened, which is that in doing a scary thing I learned a lot about myself. I got to connect with a roomful of people and witness them laugh as well as cry as I shared moments of my life. I found a musical sound that I like and am proud of. I sang my songs my way rather than trying to do what everyone else does and then telling myself I suck because I wasn't as good as the greats.

But the biggest thing I learned is that I don't particularly enjoy performing as myself. To be Brooke Shields onstage is just not comfortable for me. I don't crave being the center of attention. I know it sounds stupidly humble, but it just makes me uncomfortable. And even with all the affirming and confidence-building feedback, I realized that I felt happiest during the show when I was walking off the stage. Don't get me wrong, I love live performing, but I prefer being characters. I come alive when I'm standing in front of thousands of people wearing a wig and speaking with an accent. As myself, it's a little much. My whole life has been Brooke Brooke Brooke, and there's been this image of me as larger than life, and to be honest it can be a lot. I get a little sick of me.

That realization was a fascinating one. When you do something for so many years, you assume you like it. And I've been in the public eye for nearly my entire life. To look up and finally be able to articulate that having something be all about me isn't actually something I crave and adore took me by surprise a bit. I'd never really thought about it. And I know performers who really do crave and adore it.

When I was a teen, we would pull up to an event at a place like Studio 54 and my mom would say, "You go out first, they're not here to see me." I'd step out of the car and bulbs would flash and my name would be chanted and I'd just want to disappear. Even taking the bows at The Carlyle felt awkward and somehow indulgent. But the late, great Chita Rivera once said that bowing and taking in the applause is really about thanking the audience for giving you their time. This helps.

Am I proud to have done the show? Of course. So proud. I love that I did something that scared me more than just about anything ever has. But I was absolutely relieved when it was over. I didn't want or need the stress. The question became, however, what was it in the show that stressed me the most? I took a few weeks off and didn't sing or look at the material.

I still had the two Indianapolis performances that I'd had to reschedule, and I was honestly dreading them. But why? Well, I realized that there were two songs I hated singing, and a few jokes that never really landed. So I called my director and said, "Hey, what do you think about cutting two songs and switching them out for a couple that are more comfortable for me vocally?" He immediately agreed and said, "It's all about finding your comfort zone." (What a novel concept!) We added the first song I ever sang on a Broadway stage, "There Are Worse Things I Could Do," from *Grease*. It was the one that launched a decades-long career on Broadway for me. Then we added a Tanya Tucker song, "Delta Dawn." I switched out a few stories, tweaked some punchlines, and headed to Indiana. I could have just done the show as it was instead of paying for new orchestrations and cramming to learn new material. But I just couldn't bring myself to do it again the same way.

That's when the first miracle happened. We had a sound check and something just wasn't right. The energy was gone. We had to hire local Indianapolis band members, and although they were skilled and accomplished, it all felt lackluster. I assumed I had to just grin and bear it—the performances would all be over in two days. Instead, I was told we could let them go, with pay, and hire who we wanted. (Again, my dime, but apparently necessary.) I've been programmed to make do with less-than-optimal material and situations throughout my whole career. It didn't occur to me that I could rework whatever I wanted so that I could be my best and have fun. I had no idea I could make such big changes, but it was my show. Just because I *could* get through the earlier version didn't mean I had to. It was up to me to give myself the best chance to succeed. Except for having children, I had never felt more empowered and in control. And it seemed like such a simple fix. When I got out onstage, in front of three hundred people (versus The Carlyle's audience of one hundred), something clicked. The song and story changes, and the time off in between shows to let it all settle in—it all came together. I practically didn't recognize myself. Whose voice was that? There was a richness and a strength to it. And it didn't sound like anybody else. It was fully me.

We are, each of us, a one-woman show. But our lives are not movie montages. It's not a perfect story arc. It's messy. You are scared to do something, and you do it, and you realize you don't really want to do it after all. But you learn why. And if you choose, you change it. Or you stop doing it, because you can. You reach an age where your kids are basically cooked (but still need attention!), your relationship is what it is (but still needs to be worked on, almost daily), and it's your turn to find out what makes you happy. Maybe it's not the thing you always thought it would be, because who even had time to ask the question *what if?* We want so much to categorize and lump everything into happy endings or sad, aging or youthful, this or that. But life is not binary, and we are not just one thing. We are all these things at the same time, and that doesn't make us a contradiction in terms, it just means we are interesting and multidimensional.

Society wants to lump all of us "aging" women in one category they know what to do with because it feels more palatable. *Here is a tale as old as time, a story we can understand!* But perhaps the power comes from continuing to confuse, or at least surprise, those who think they know us best—whether that's our families and friends or the gatekeepers of our media and culture. Our stories cannot be foisted upon us. We own the narrative.

2

Not Backing Down, Not Backing Out

A LESSON IN CONFIDENCE

Writing *Down Came the Rain* was not easy, to put it mildly. While I've learned to have no shame about experiencing postpartum depression (about one in eight women experience symptoms[1]), it was not exactly something I was proud of, especially in 2005, when it was far less openly discussed than it is today.

Rowan was born in 2003. A year later, with the help of medication and therapy, I was coming out of the fog of PPD and getting healthier. One day, I was at lunch with my then-agent, John Kimble, with whom I'd been honest about my struggles. I had no choice really, because it had been a difficult year and had affected my work. "You need to write about this experience," he said.

Not unlike the show at The Carlyle, I wasn't interested. I said, "Nobody needs to hear another celebrity lamenting how hard things have been for them. Why would anyone care that I was sad?"

"This is a real condition," John said. "It's happening to so many women and nobody is talking about it and the medical industry barely recognizes it. All we hear about are the women who kill their babies." Postpartum depression exists on a spectrum, but because only the extreme cases make headlines there is a real shame and stigma surrounding it. John added, "You can help change that!" I have to give him credit—not all men understand and take this condition seriously, but he saw the value in a book that shared my truth, and also the opportunity it could provide for others to heal. Even before I signed on to the idea, John understood that by my shedding light on this issue, real change—both in public perception as well as legislative policy—might be possible. He positioned it to me as my social responsibility. Well, that was all I needed to hear.

My biggest fear at the time was becoming a sob story—boohoo, poor Brooke Shields. I really didn't want or need pity. For so long I'd felt guilty that I wasn't maternal enough, or scared that I would never bond with my daughter, and I certainly didn't want public opinion confirming that. Women have been having babies since the dawn of time, I thought, so what the fuck is my problem? Maybe I'd had it too good for too long and this was my punishment for decades of good fortune. The universe balancing the scales. (Did I mention I was raised Catholic?)

But in therapy I learned about the biology of PPD, and about what was happening to my mind as well as the rest of my body. Information about PPD is more readily available today but was hard to come by twenty years ago. I realized that "toughen up and fight it out" was not a coping strategy, as much as I willed it to be. And if *I* hadn't known any of this, as someone with plenty of privilege and resources and quality medical providers, maybe John had a point. Maybe I could help other women or, more important to me at the time, help my daughter. I knew she might one day have babies and could experience something similar, and I didn't want her to be made to feel faulty or broken or bad or less than as a mother. I didn't want my shame to inhibit what could be a valuable teaching moment. So we went to a publishing company, pitched the book to a couple of executives, and I had my first book deal.

Down Came the Rain came out on May 3, 2005. About a month and a half later, Tom Cruise famously went on the *Today* show, ostensibly to promote his film *War of the Worlds*. But in the process he disparaged me, referring to my use of antidepressants and that I spoke publicly about it as "dangerous." I was, according to Tom, spreading misinformation. An interesting opinion, coming from someone without ovaries.

Tom and I had known each other for twenty years at that point. He had a small part in *Endless Love*, and he always had a fondness for my mother because she had looked out for him on set. We'd come up in our industry around the same time, and we'd only ever gotten along. His attack left me gobsmacked. (All of a sudden I'm British, but I so love that word.) However, this was a couple of months after he'd jumped on Oprah's couch. He was surprising everyone.

I was never one to find myself in a public feud. The news of my and Andre's divorce made headlines, but we didn't try our case in the court of public opinion. It happened relatively quickly and quietly. Had Tom taken a public swing at me before I became a mother, I probably would have stayed quiet. I would have ignored his ridiculous rant. I might have been content to sit back while this very famous man hijacked my experience to advance his own (deluded) agenda. I would have been satisfied that his behavior would speak for itself.

Unlucky for Tom, however, his appearance on the *Today* show took place almost exactly a month after my fortieth birthday. Sitting quietly and letting myself be attacked might have been my approach a decade earlier—I might have even regretted sharing my story or felt insecure that maybe my career was stalling while a powerful male movie star was singling me out, sure that I'd never stand a chance in that fight—but now I was emboldened by life experience. At forty, I was growing into my self-confidence. I had begun to shift my thought process from "everyone knows better than I do" to "I know myself best," and so instead of letting myself turn into a punching bag, I swung back.

On July 1, a few days after Tom's *Today* show appearance, I published an op-ed in the *New York Times*—"War of Words"—in response to his comments. "I'm going to take a wild guess and say that Mr. Cruise has never suffered from postpartum depression," I wrote, before using data to refute his claims about how I should have used vitamins and exercise to combat my depression. I should point out that my publicist at the time told me not to dignify his comments with a response, which only infuriated me more. I wasn't dignifying anything! I was sticking up for myself, and for women who were suffering, against irrational and dangerous comments from an unschooled actor who was speaking way out of his depth. (I fired that publicist, by the way.)

I chose to write the op-ed because I knew that if I spoke out in an interview, rather than in writing, my words would be chopped up and crafted into whatever sound bites the journalists wanted. That had happened to me plenty in my career, especially when I commented on my personal life or mentioned other actors. (Once, in the 1980s, a journalist asked my opinion about Jodie Foster. The question was something like, "What do you think about Jodie Foster's success since she's respected and you've traveled such a different path?" *Uh, thanks.* I went on to say how much I, too, respected Jodie and how talented and formidable and brilliant she was. But did I look at her and think, *What about me?* No. Well, here's the quote the journalist used: "I look at her and think, what about me?" It made me look so bratty and jealous, and I knew that I could never again fully trust journalists to quote me with accuracy.)

It's possible that Tom chose me as his target because he thought I'd simply take the hit. Despite gracing covers of magazines and being celebrated for my looks, I didn't have a ton of confidence in my younger years. Maybe it was *because* I was celebrated primarily for my looks. I didn't feel like people took the rest of me—my intellect and my talent, in particular—very seriously. And I was never really encouraged to have strong opinions or to use my voice. I was taught to be a people pleaser. "Everyone's a fan," my mother would tell me. There was not one person I didn't sign an autograph for or take a picture with if they asked, even in a huge group of people. There was not one piece of fan mail that wasn't opened and responded to with an autographed photo. The underlying message was always: give the people what they want. My success relied on my popularity, and my popularity relied on saying yes to practically everything. Discovering what I wanted wasn't as important as delivering what everyone else wanted. I was an easy mark for a powerful man.

My op-ed sparked outrage at Tom (never my intention) and spurred discussions on the reality and prevalence of postpartum depression. Suddenly there was an opportunity to give voice to the hardships of women and families who had suffered as I had. It was really one of the first times I had stood up for myself in a public forum with a deep sense of conviction that what I was doing was right. For so long, I had deferred to my mother, who always seemed to have the answers I didn't. I relied on her to dictate my opinion on almost everything. (I have a vivid memory of eating a bowl of French onion soup as a kid and asking my mom, "Do I like this?") Throughout much of my life I internalized the idea that others knew what was best for me. This served me well because it labeled me a "good girl," but it was a while before I learned to trust my own instincts and realize that I know myself better than anybody else does.

It took me a long time to see how damaging this mindset was, and to realize how pervasive it is for girls, and even young women, to struggle with confidence. A survey commissioned by Katty Kay and Claire Shipman, authors of *The Confidence Code* and *The Confidence Code for Girls*, found that between the ages of eight and fourteen, girls' confidence drops by 30 percent.[2] Before age twelve, there is no difference in the confidence levels of girls and boys. After age twelve, confidence doesn't match up again until around age fifty, if at all. The survey also found that girls' confidence that other people like them falls 46 percent between their tween and teen years, and that girls are 18 percent less likely than boys to describe themselves as confident. (They are, however, more likely to use words like "anxious," "worried," and "stressed.")

It's not at all accurate to say that I woke up one morning and my insecurities disappeared in an instant. But right around age forty, I began to tire of looking externally for answers and validation. It was exhausting quite honestly. The dormant part of me that could trust myself and my opinions and desires started rearing its head. Oh the audacity! For me, there was also an element of wanting to model confidence for my girls, which really pushed me to fake it till I made it—but research shows that, children or not, women in their forties and fifties report feeling more confident as they age. One survey of American women over the age of thirty-five found that 64 percent say they feel more confident now than in their younger years.[3] Another survey of an even older cohort found that 59 percent of women over fifty said they feel more confident as they've aged.[4] And yet another study found that women report having significantly lower confidence than men until age fifty, at which point the confidence levels of each gender finally align.[5]

I suppose it's important to take a step back here. What is confidence, anyway? What does it mean to have it or not have it? I spoke to *Confidence Code* coauthor Katty Kay, who shared that confidence is often misunderstood. "Women have for so long thought about confidence and wondered, *Do you have to be a jerk to be confident? Is the confident person the one who speaks the loudest and longest? The one who has the most swagger?* If that's what confidence is understood to be, it's no wonder women don't find it appealing," she said. But I was one of those women. For a long time, I thought confidence was the belief that you were great. I thought it was about believing in your opinions and talent without caring about other people's input. Confidence was black or white, but also a catch-22. If I had too much, I was arrogant; not enough, I was weak.

What confidence really is, according to psychologists, is a belief in your abilities and in your capacity to overcome challenges. It's not about thinking you are better than anyone else, and, in fact, psychologists say that the people with the healthiest confidence are those who can admit when they don't know something, because they have, yes, *confidence* in their ability to learn it. Kay told me that when she and her coauthor Claire Shipman were researching their book, the best definition of "confidence" came from a psychologist at Ohio State University, who told them that "confidence is the stuff that turns thought into action." It's when your perception of your ability is aligned with your actual ability, so that you're willing to try new or scary things because you know you can handle them.

It's one thing to understand confidence intellectually, but it's another thing to truly *feel* it. For most of us, confidence ebbs and flows—there are times when we feel fully empowered, and other times when we struggle to find our voice. Kay told me that we can work on developing confidence by actively pushing our boundaries. "When you overcome hurdles, when you try things that are hard and new—that is how you grow your confidence,"

Kay says. "It doesn't come from people telling you you're great or reading a great review. It's by trying things that are hard for you. I see it as a wall made of bricks, and every time you do something difficult and overcome it, or even fail and but keep going anyway, you can put another brick in your wall."

Not only do women gain confidence with age—but we also do so at a higher clip than our male peers. While both genders see an increase in confidence over the years, women see a "steadier, sharper climb," according to research.[6] I find this fascinating. What makes women, who suffer from lower confidence than men in our younger years, surpass them as we age? I guess "because we're fucking awesome" isn't a good-enough answer, though there's plenty of truth to it. Experts say it has something to do with caring less about what others think than men do, which is tied to what Kay describes as "volatile confidence." When your confidence is dependent on external validation—compliments, positive reviews of your work, "likes" on social media—that good feeling can be taken away just as quickly as it was bestowed. It's volatile. Younger people are more prone to embracing this type of confidence, Kay says. As are men. But as women age, and overcome more hard things, they've built a larger bank of confidence that becomes more solid.

Biology may also play a part, or so Kay speculates. "We know that estrogen does many wonderful things, but it can also drive some of the people-pleasing we see in teenage girls," she says. "As women age, head into menopause, and produce less estrogen, it stands to reason that the desire to please declines. I've heard doctors say women become less nurturing as they hit menopause, but there's a more positive way to see that: we care less what people think of us. We become less perfectionist. All that helps boost our confidence."

Kay, who is not only a four-time bestselling author but also

39

a mother of four and the US correspondent for BBC Studios and a contributor to MSNBC, was fifty-nine when we spoke. She said her research findings about women and confidence were reinforced by personal experience. "I would say my confidence in my ability is higher than it's ever been," she told me. "In my fifties, I started to trust my instincts. When I was thirty, I would never have thought I could do the things that I'm doing now." Kay says she has banked enough confidence to know that if she takes on something new, she will probably make it work. "And that's really freeing. It allows me to do things that are in line with my values and turn down opportunities that are not, and thus set myself up for success."

For me, the journey to becoming more confident was also about wanting to feel less stressed-out and worried all the time. There came a day when I was simply tired of judging myself and feeling like I wasn't enough. I was over the angst. I didn't want to be mean to myself anymore, and I started to wonder where I got the idea that I needed to be perfect at everything anyway. *What would it feel like in my body if I told myself I'm smart, I'm talented, I'm strong, I'm beautiful, I'm a good person and friend?* I asked myself. *What if I just assumed I was good enough as is?* Turns out, it's liberating! I felt like the Stay Puft Marshmallow Man in *Ghostbusters*, filled to near bursting with belief in myself. I got all New Yorker about it, walking around with a "try to fuck with me, I dare you" attitude. (Once the bravado of newfound strength settled in a bit, the actual relief of no longer beating myself up took over.)

In the late 1990s, my career was in a slump. I needed work, and we needed money, so I signed a deal to promote a weight-loss product in Japan. Twice a day I had to go inside this weird chamber for an hour, where I was tightly wrapped up in something like cellophane and basically dehydrated so they could say the product worked. (The company has since folded, big surprise.) I was claustrophobic and going out of my mind, so my then-bodyguard gave me a set of self-help tapes—this was in the Walkman era—to help me pass the time and stave off the claustrophobia. At one point I remember listening to a discussion of how the brain is a computer. Its job is to find an answer to any question it is posed. If you ask negative questions (*Why don't I have a better body?* or *Why don't I have a boyfriend?*) your brain will come up with answers (*You have no self-control* or *You're too bossy*), and it will think it's done its job. All these years later, that tape sticks with me. I remember thinking, *Wow, what would happen if I started asking better, more positive, questions, like why do people like being around me? Why am I successful?* Once again, the brain comes up with answers—*You're good company* or *You work hard and you're talented*—and suddenly you have a new narrative.

I'll admit, the increase in confidence—or the willingness to *choose* confidence—has been my favorite part about this stage of life. I used to back out of rooms because I thought my ass was too big. Today? Who has time for that? I'm a grown (-ass) adult woman, I don't need to be backing myself through doorways (especially because I've become somewhat spatially challenged and even more clumsy these days). I used to avoid looking in the mirror whenever I was in public, because I never wanted to appear vain. But then, at dance class, I would fall on my face. My dance teacher would yell at me: "Shields! If you don't spot yourself in the mirror, you'll never find your center!"

I used to go to parties and find myself doing dishes at the end of the night not just to be polite but because I felt I somehow had to earn my invitation. (Even just reading this over, I can see that it's nutty.) Now I arrive, say "thank you for having me," and enjoy myself because I deserve to be there. *Glamour* recently described me as being in my "fuck-it era." It was a cute headline and a good article, but I think it's less about throwing your hands up and saying *who cares* and more about believing that if there's something you want to say, it inherently has value.

I won't pretend I wasn't scared when I responded to Tom Cruise's antics. Of course I was. Cancel culture wasn't yet a thing, but when you're in the public eye and you speak out, you get concerned, not unreasonably, that the media will pummel you, and that the fans whose respect you've worked so hard to earn will follow suit. Or you worry that you'll be painted as a "hysterical woman" (because, of course, that's also often what happens). In that particular instance, speaking up was made easier because I wasn't sticking up just for myself; I was sticking up for women and mothers everywhere. If I *didn't* say something, what kind of a woman was I? And because it went well—because my response was supported and because, frankly, all the attention worked in favor of women—I was able to derive even more confidence. It won't always go swimmingly, but when you stand up for yourself when you believe you must, and it feels good and doesn't blow up in your face, you start to wonder . . . where else can I take this approach? Not in a defensive way necessarily (much of the time you really shouldn't engage with the haters), but I could at the very least reconsider my people-pleasing tendencies and say no to the opportunities that weren't right for me. I could trust that I knew myself best, and not defer to everyone else just because I perceived they had more power.

At a certain age, whatever fear you have about saying no or standing up for yourself or speaking out really is mitigated by caring less about what others think. You want to do something scary, and you hesitate, and then you think: *What's the worst that could*

42

happen? Being afraid is normal, and fear doesn't just evaporate as you get older, but it can be a motivator. Eventually it's coupled with an ability to ask yourself, *What am I afraid of? How bad could it be? Why not try?*

So I practiced. I spoke up more on my own behalf. I trusted my instincts. If they'd gotten me this far, they must have some value. I said no to things I didn't want to do, which felt terrifying and defiant but also revelatory. This sometimes came as a shock to others, who'd grown to expect one thing of me and suddenly had to readjust. Take my husband, who tends to offer his opinion on what I should and shouldn't do in my life, whether I've asked for it or not. He wants to protect me, I know. His advice stems from a place of love because he's seen the way the media can treat a famous person. He might call it "guiding" or "helping" me. But at some point I had to say, as kindly as I could, *Could you stop? I can handle myself.* If you've been in a relationship dynamic for so many years, your evolution might come as a shock to the other person, be it a spouse or kids or friends or family, since no one warned them it was coming. It's not a bait and switch, but any adjustment is hard, especially for the people who've settled into expecting one thing from you and—surprise!—find that you're still changing. But a lot can come of reminding others that you're still evolving. You can even ask how it makes them feel, while gently reminding them that if they're uncomfortable, that's something *they'll* need to deal with. You can't be static in order to accommodate someone else's feelings.

I practiced speaking up and saying no at work, too. I'm not what anyone would label a diva, and have never aspired to be, but in the past I've taken a "put your head down and do the work" approach to any job I've been offered. It's a trait that has served me well, but it has also prevented me, at times, from considering whether I actually believed in the work, or even wanted

to be doing it. In 2014, I signed a contract with the Hallmark
Channel for sixteen movies. I'd completed only three when I
realized I had to renegotiate. I'd been hired, I was told, to help
change the face of the network. They wanted me to be funny
and bring more comedy to their offerings, but as filming progressed on each of the Flower Shop Mysteries—the franchise I
was hired to headline—all the humor had evaporated. My mom
used to tell me that work generates work. "Nothing is beneath
you," she'd say. But there's something to be said for earning the
right to be particular and discerning. Not everything is for everyone, and there is absolutely nothing wrong with the Hallmark
Channel—God knows it has a huge fan base—but it was not the
future I wanted for my career. I'm never against hard work, but
I am now a believer in only saying yes to work that serves me. I
realized that I could make a living with other opportunities (that
I enjoyed more and required less time away from my family),
and I simply could not do *thirteen* more films that were not
what I was promised and felt completely wrong for me. So I
quit. I definitely surprised some people, and in plenty of ways I
surprised myself. I certainly would never have done that in my
twenties. Back then it was "you're so lucky, you're so lucky; be
thankful, be thankful." Now I could tell myself, *Yes, luck plays
a part in most careers but so does talent, intelligence, and strong
work ethic.* Maybe I've earned the right to say "no, this is not
acceptable to me" and move on.

I saw a study recently[7] that was inspired by the author, a business school professor, noticing that her students' evaluations of
her teaching declined in her forties, even as her experience and
expertise and confidence grew. In the resulting research, she
found that women are perceived as "less warm" as they age and
thus are judged more harshly. It reminded me of what many of us
already know: if you're a man who is forthright, you're a leader.

A woman, you're a bitch. When men exude confidence, it's not only expected but admired, whereas when we do, it's met with shock and disdain. It was a reminder that while women are more confident as we mature, the world is just catching up. We age into a newfound belief in ourselves, but outside reactions tend to be something along the lines of "What got into her?!?" rather than "Good for her!"

For a long time, whenever I complained about this double standard, I was pretty much met with a shrug and a response of "that's just how the world works." And that may be true, but now I know it's not how *I'm* going to work.

Of course, I still have insecurities. But I feel good about more than I don't. I am confident about the way my brain processes information, about my body's strength and its ability to heal. I've raised amazing children. I like my long hair. I believe I'm a very talented comedic actress. And it's still hard for me to say all this without a disclaimer—"don't think I'm arrogant!"—but I do it anyway, because it's about time. I make the choice, every day, not to let my insecurities dictate my behavior or my choices. To act from a place of confidence. After all, we've gotten this far. We must have done something right.

Eventually Tom Cruise apologized to me. Not publicly, which would have been the right thing to do, but he came to my house and said he was sorry and that he felt cornered by Matt Lauer and that he attacked me, basically, because he could. It wasn't the world's best apology, but it's what he was capable of, and I accepted it. (The crazy thing was that by this time our daughters—his first, my second—had been born, and on the same day. And, get this . . . in the same hospital, in the same room. I remember walking into the hospital, ready to have Grier, with my head down—we had a decoy car and were focused on avoiding the paparazzi—but as I entered I noticed all these people walking in the opposite direction. They were leaving the hospital with umbrellas, clearly shielding themselves from view. I got to my room and looked out the window and saw hordes of news vans and photographers and thought, *Damn, can't they leave me alone to have this experience?* Well, imagine my embarrassment when a nurse whispered that the fuss outside was not, in fact, for me but for Tom and Katie and their freshly birthed baby girl. I learned later that it was the new parents and their entourage who were leaving the hospital's loading dock as we were going in.)

The whole controversy, or Cruise-gate, as we began calling it, ultimately worked in my favor and in favor of women everywhere. Tom didn't have a leg to stand on, and his ignorance on the issue inspired women to get on their soapboxes and scream for their rights and their bodies. Having a famous movie star attacking my journey brought attention to it. I testified in front of Congress. In New Jersey, a law was passed requiring doctors to educate expectant mothers about PPD and to screen them for depression at postpartum visits. I wasn't laughed at or made to feel guilty, I was applauded. And these external outcomes, while meaningful, were secondary to the realization that I am my own best spokesperson. Today, I know what is best for me, and I feel certain that trusting myself—and prioritizing myself—will only benefit me. It's nice when other people appreciate you, but these days, the biggest rush comes from valuing myself. From saying, *Actually, I believe in myself, and I'm proud of me.*

Who knew, in a career where I starred as a prostitute at age eleven, where I played a mother at age fifteen, that valuing myself at fifty-nine would be my most provocative choice?

3

Character Study

GIVING YOURSELF THE CREDIT YOU DESERVE

was standing backstage at the Eccles Theater in Park City as the credits began to roll on the screening of *Pretty Baby: Brooke Shields*, the documentary about my life and career that premiered at Sundance in January 2023. I was scheduled to participate in a Q&A with director Lana Wilson after the screening, but from where I was standing, it appeared that most of the audience was getting on their feet and preparing to leave the theater.

Oh, too bad, I thought. *I was hoping some people would stick around for the aftershow.*

Suddenly, Ali Wentworth, my dear friend and executive producer on the film, was pushing me onto the stage. "They aren't leaving, silly, they're applauding!" she said. It was a standing ovation—a wild round of applause. I was honestly confused. I was getting applauded for . . . what, exactly? Surviving?

The idea for the documentary came from Ali herself. She and I first became friends in 2016, and she always seemed to harbor some shock at how "normal" I had turned out. "I can't believe you're not in rehab, much less that you're alive" she'd say when we chatted about the early years of my career. It's certainly true that plenty of celebrities who rose to fame as children have experienced different, sometimes tragic, trajectories. The truth is, I absolutely understand the urge to shave your head, smash a car window with an umbrella, and say fuck you to all the craziness. To punch a paparazzo. The hounding is constant from the moment you leave your house, and that can really mess with a person. Ali and I discussed all this and I would tell her that I had to make the choice for myself. I had to fight for normalcy. I never believed all the hype about me, or that I was better than anyone else. I just always wanted to fit in and have a real life. I've been working a long time and I've seen plenty of people get destroyed by this business. My attitude has always been, *I will not let them win.* Still, it would have been easy to get sucked into the mayhem and madness. As it happened, my decision—no, my *insistence*—that I not become a statistic was a bigger rebellion against the system than any drug addiction or partying would have ever been.

In 2021, Ali and her husband, George Stephanopoulos, started a production company called BedBy8, and they approached me with the idea of creating a documentary on my life as their first project. It was flattering if a bit humbling—*Have I lived long enough to warrant a documentary? Have I reached the stage in my career where I am being relegated to being the subject of a "where are they now" or an* E! True Hollywood Story? (I'd been approached about documentaries before and the pitches were always slanted in that direction.) But Ali and George said they wanted this film to shed light on the objectification of young women in this country, and, for better or worse, my career was the perfect on-ramp to tell that larger story.

I wouldn't have said yes to just anyone, but I trusted Ali and George. They are both incredibly smart, and I knew they would never exploit me. Plus, they hoped to bring on Emmy Award–winning director Lana Wilson, who had directed such acclaimed documentaries as *The Departure* (about punk-rocker-turned-Buddhist-priest Ittetsu Nemoto), *After Tiller* (about abortion providers), and the Taylor Swift doc *Miss Americana*. I knew that she was not only brilliant but also that she would find a resonating and relatable way to tell a bigger, more important story than simply one of an actress growing up in the public eye. Honestly, because her most recent film was with Taylor Swift, I was surprised she accepted the gig! But when she did, I knew she wouldn't want to make a salacious exposé but a smart piece of commentary on our society.

About ten years ago, I digitized my archives—every interview, appearance, magazine cover, and print ad I had done back when nothing was memorialized online was now on a thumb drive that I kept in my office. The day I met Lana, I handed that drive over to her. In retrospect, I don't think she'd fully grasped the scope of my career until she began combing through it all. After all, she was born in 1983. She wasn't even alive when *Pretty Baby* and *Blue Lagoon* played in theaters, or when my Calvin Klein ads were on TV. But what most impressed Lana, she later shared, wasn't so much the magnitude of my career but my poise as a little girl in the limelight—in particular, the way I conducted my-self in interviews. When I was young, journalists and TV hosts interrogated me about my mom. Everyone had an opinion about my mother and the way she managed my career, and for what-ever reason, they thought it appropriate to share that opinion with an eleven-, twelve-, thirteen-year-old girl on national TV. I was fierce in my defense of her, and I resented being forced into the position of having to do so. In the end, I think Lana did an amazing job with the footage, and she not only painted a clear picture of what it was like to be me but also how my experience was representative of how we as a society treated—and maybe still treat—young girls and women.

Despite having commissioned the digital archive of all my

interviews and appearances, it wasn't until I sat in the screening room to view the finished and cut film that I watched any of the clips from my past. That was the first time I allowed myself to pause and reflect on all I've survived, and honestly, I don't think I could have handled doing this project any earlier in my life. I had never looked back, only forward. It was always "what's next?" because I wanted to reach the next stage of my career or the next stage in my personal life. As young women, we aren't encouraged to sit still so much as we are expected to put one foot in front of the other and keep it all together and satisfy other people. As we become adults, our job becomes to help those who rely on us to stay afloat. I never really reflected on my own story. Even my book *There Was a Little Girl* was written as a meditation on my mother, and my relationship with her, more than it was a reflection on myself. I could only stomach that kind of examination if it was in the context of my connection to someone else. Spending too much time thinking about "everything Brooke" seemed self-indulgent and, quite honestly, boring.

All that changed with the *Pretty Baby* documentary. Working on a documentary about my life obviously forced some introspection, but while watching the film, I too marveled at myself as a little girl. I never fully realized how desperately I wanted to do the right thing for the people around me. I hadn't known how much I was also trying to fight for my truths and figure out who I was, independent of public opinion or my mother. There's one interview that didn't make the final cut, but in it, a reporter asks me, at about age thirteen, the same question over and over again. I keep answering the same way, and when I do, this woman tries again to trip me up, just phrasing the question differently, insistent on getting me to answer it the way *she* wanted me to answer. I finally said, "I'm sorry, ma'am, but I don't think you want my answer, because I keep answering you and I don't have a different answer—this is my truth." Watching that clip four decades later, I was in awe of that little girl on-screen. *I had that in me? I* thought. *At that age??* But over time that sense of self-possession got eaten away. What happened in my teens and twenties and thirties to obliterate it? It took me years to regain that level of confidence and assertiveness, but I watched my younger self with a sense of pride that there had always been a measure of resilience in me. And much like my friend Ali, I marveled that I've been able to arrive where I am today. I survived all of it. I've been in this business for six decades, and I'm still standing. I didn't expect to be as proud as I am to have weathered my existence, but I'm even more proud of having done so with strong healthy friendships and a solid family intact.

Most of us don't get to watch documentaries capturing our life stories, I get that. But we've all been through stuff. If you've made it to forty or fifty or sixty, it's inevitable that you've lived through conflict and loss. You've survived moments, or months, or maybe even years that felt unbearable. As a woman, you've existed in a society that undermines you at every turn yet still demands the world from you. And despite all this, you've made it. You have so much to show for yourself! You might even have your own version of archives, from old photos to letters and diary entries that are memorialized in a drawer in your nightstand or a box under the bed. You could look back and pat yourself on the back for making it through, but I'm willing to bet you haven't spent much time doing that. I'd venture to guess that you aren't giving yourself enough credit. If you're anything like me, you probably credit everyone else for your success, or your survival, while shrugging off any of the accolades that you most definitely deserve.

I've been going to the same therapist for thirty-five years. She's seen me through, well, *a lot*. Career highs and lows, a very public marriage, divorce, remarriage, kids, postpartum depression, motherhood, the loss of a best friend to suicide, the loss of both my parents, my kids leaving the nest . . . she's witnessed my entire adulthood. One day I was talking to her about the documentary and this general "how did you turn out so normal?" reaction that many people have (I'm not saying they're *rooting* for me to be a statistic or cliché, but it remains such a shock to people that I am not a mess), and I guess I was doing my usual song and dance about all the external reasons I turned out okay: I had loving parents, I was privileged, I was pretty, I was educated, I didn't grow up in L.A. so I knew a world outside Hollywood. I hadn't thought of my survival as something to applaud or be proud of. The alternative was simply never an option as far as I was concerned. Some form of normalcy was always the focus and the goal, and I wasn't going to let myself not have that.

My therapist looked me dead in the eyes and said, "When are you going to allow yourself to see that your survival is a result of your individual character? You attribute everything to everybody else, but nobody pulled you from going off the rails. Something inside you—some strength that can't be taught—wouldn't allow yourself to be beaten. When are you going to give yourself a little credit?" She reminded me that I did okay under less-than-ideal circumstances. Sure, I was famous, and I had earned money, but I was also the daughter of an alcoholic for whom I felt responsible from an incredibly young age, and I was under constant scrutiny by the news media and the public, who felt they owned me. In addition, the entire world seemed to constantly be implying that my real currency lay solely in my looks. (Okay, maybe not the most optimal of circumstances for normalcy.) But for some reason I kept fighting to stay afloat and find my balance.

You won't be surprised to hear by now that this tendency to not give ourselves enough credit is much more common in women. It's researched most often in business settings. One study found that women underestimate their job performance ratings by 11 percent.[1] Another study found that women consistently rated their performance on a test lower than men rated themselves, even though both groups had the same average score *and* these women were told outright that their self-evaluation would affect their pay and potential for promotion.[2] It's not hard to extrapolate these findings to other groups—mothers certainly don't give themselves enough credit for all that they do. Women, in general, no matter our life story . . . we're so hard on ourselves! One survey of two thousand women found that we criticize ourselves at least eight times a day, and frankly that seems to be a pretty low number. And we all—male or female—suffer from negativity bias, as our brains are wired to focus on the bad over the good. When we reflect on our pasts, we tend to give our mistakes far more weight than our successes.

But consider this: looking kindly on your accomplishments and celebrating your wins can have a significant impact on your psychological health. Researchers say acknowledging your accomplishments can help boost your mood and increase motivation and productivity. Self-compassion, or treating yourself like you would a friend (building yourself up instead of tearing yourself down), decreases stress and increases resilience and well-being, especially as you age.[3] Not only do we deserve credit for doing all the hard things we've already done (and we have done so many! All of us!), but giving ourselves credit also sets us up to do even more hard things. Because remember, we've got time: if you are a woman reading this at age forty, your life expectancy is another forty-one years.[4] You're not nearing the end, you're only halfway there!

Reflecting on your life and giving yourself credit for all you've done is not the same as living in the past. That sort of attitude helps no one. No matter how much I wish I'd appreciated my youthful looks and young body when I had them—that I'd said "good on you, kid" a bit more than I did—there's no part of me that wants to go back there or do any of it over again. I truly feel like I got through the hard years and now I'm at the place where I get to have fun and be creative because there is no preconceived notion of what this stage looks like. It's fucking exciting! I love knowing where I came from, but now I get to mix it up a little.

After the documentary premiered on Hulu, I went on the *Today* show to discuss it with Hoda Kotb and Jenna Bush Hager. Jenna asked me if there was anything in my past that I wish had never happened. "What would you erase?" she asked, referring to the entirety of my life story. It's a big question. There were a lot of hard times, including some, like a sexual assault, that I revealed for the first time in the film. But I told her the truth—I would only erase my mother's alcoholism, which was a constant source of agony for me. But honestly, even that made me stronger and more prepared to navigate human behavior. And truly everything else I've survived not only made me resilient but also gave me perspective and put me in the position I'm in today to tell my story and advocate for other women. As clichéd as it may seem, every challenge allowed me to grow and learn. Spending most of my life under public scrutiny has acclimated me to receive whatever criticism or judgment that comes my way with a sort of "bring it on" attitude. (Or should I call it armor?) It may seem unfortunate that I had to earn such an attitude by being attacked by the press and even the public, but I really did become a resilient woman, and now I wear that attitude with pride.

I'm learning to let go of any regret for things that were truly out of my control. When we're younger, regret has some value—it can encourage us to make better choices. But as we age, the ability to *let go* of regret is tied to both emotional and physical health. After all, regret is about the past. Becoming mired in thoughts about events that happened decades ago robs us of the time and focus we can invest in activities and relationships that bring us joy. These days I'm more interested in preventing new regrets. Studies show that as we hit our forties, fifties, and sixties, most of our regrets are tied to inaction rather than action.[5] We regret all that stuff we *didn't* do, the roads we didn't take, the opportunities we let slip by. I want to keep taking chances and challenging myself (see: chapter 1). I want to embrace the idea of feeling the fear and doing it anyway. This is our time to take the opportunities we don't want to miss out on, rather than sit back because we're worried how it will turn out or what others will think.

That being said, I am also very much okay with accepting my limits. Now, I want to clarify that acceptance is not defeat, or resignation, which I think of as feeling tired and beaten down by all you've been through. Acceptance is also knowing that you can't or don't want to do something, or even that you've aged out of it. (Maybe your body just doesn't bend that way anymore, or perhaps staying up until the wee hours of the night—which was exciting decades ago—no longer holds much appeal.) A few years ago some women I was hanging out with at the beach told me they had started surfing on Sundays. Keep in mind that I have never wanted to learn to surf. I'd love to know how to surf, to *have done it*, but I didn't want to go through the labor of learning the sport. I'm also very afraid of deep dark water (analyze that any way you want). But for some reason, when these women asked if I wanted to join them, I pictured stand-up paddleboarding. You know, a giant board. A paddle. The ability to sit comfortably on your butt and coast if need be. That sort of thing.

When I showed up on the beach at the assigned time, however, I saw a giant pile of wet suits and surfboards in front of me. I didn't want to look like a wimp, so I went for it. Put on a suit, grabbed a board. With surfing, you're supposed to start by paddling as hard as you can with the tip of your board aimed directly at oncoming waves. That in itself is terrifying. But I wouldn't give up. I would conquer my fear! I refused to fail. I started meeting these women every Sunday. The more I surfed, the more frustrated and exhausted I became. I was always happiest when the session was over and I could peel the gross, too-tight rubber contraption off my now-freezing body. Then, one day, I actually did pop up. I caught a wave and even managed to stand and extend my ride to the next rolling wave and all the way to shallow water. I got the vibe! I understood the freedom and exhilaration! *This is it*, I thought. I am now a surfer. Well, I was never able to do it again. Soon I couldn't even paddle out without feeling paralyzed. The waves coming at me just felt too intimidating. The final time I met the ladies, I fell off my board and felt the tug of the rope on my ankle, which is the signal that the board is moving away from you. I stood up just in time for the board to come crashing down on my head. I got a concussion, and still I begged my instructor to let me go back out there. Of course, I was told to go nowhere but back to the beach.

Once safely at home with a nice-size lump on my head, it occurred to me that *oh yeah, I am not enjoying this*. I wanted to say I could do it, and maybe become more comfortable in deep water. But my fear never subsided, and there was very little reward for me in any of it. I watched the other women get so excited by these group lessons and I saw them riding the waves easily and they just seemed so happy. I wanted to feel what they felt. But did

I actually *like* surfing? Not really. I also didn't particularly like the feeling of not being good at it. And that's perfectly okay! I've accomplished my fair share in life. I've survived decades of shit thrown my way, and if I don't want to add surfing to that list of things I've overcome, it doesn't mean I've failed.

What's interesting is that surviving all the stuff we do in order to get to this more mature chapter is what makes us happier as we age. Laura Carstensen, a professor of psychology and founding director of the Stanford Center on Longevity, has found that people over fifty report more positive emotions and fewer negative ones—and the negative ones they do report are less intense. But it's not as simple as "older people are happier." As she said in a 2021 interview with NPR's *On Point*: "Older people have more mixed emotions. They're more likely to experience joy with a tear in the eye than younger people are. We see a kind of a savoring and an appreciation, that's what captures the emotional experience. It is not a uniform, simplistic, happy." It's a better, richer happy! The reason for this, she says, is experience: "Older people are affected by terrible things, just as younger people are. But they come to that with experience, and they come to that with a perspective. . . . There's a sense when something negative happens that you've been here before, and that this time will pass." That we can handle life with so much more resolve is absolutely one of the best parts of being in middle age. Having lived for five or six decades, we are no longer like our kids, for whom every day is the best day ever or absolute worst day ever. My daughters, for example, live at both extremes. I'll watch the pendulum swing so ferociously from one end to the other that I marvel it doesn't do a 360 and take off like a rocket. For Grier especially, every negative incident is the worst in the world. Sometimes I'll listen to her talk about her days, and my heart just breaks for her. She is such a deeply feeling person and has beautifully high standards for how she wants to behave, but she expects her friends and the world to act accordingly. And she is constantly disappointed. When that happens, I no longer try to fix things or rationalize with her. It just escalates the drama. I listen and wait until the dust settles, and then maybe, just maybe, I inquire if she'd like to discuss the issue further. Usually by that point she just shrugs it off and moves on.

For me, nothing is all good or all bad anymore. The nuance is clearer. When things are hard, I know they won't be hard for long. "This too shall pass" is a phrase that makes even more sense to me as I get older. The hard times eventually are behind us. As are the good ones! With maturity, we have enough experience to see and appreciate the complexity of our experiences, and feel more joy overall. That's powerful stuff.

I've made peace with exactly where I am in my life at this moment. Not just peace with it—I welcome it! I'm also looking forward to seeing what will come next. But the only way to really embrace a new beginning is to be okay with closing the previous chapter. By looking back, saying "I did that!" and taking all you've learned, for better and worse, and using it as tools for the next phase. I recognize this is not easy, and it takes reflection and work—both of which can be scary. But it is so liberating, trust me. Working on the documentary was the first time in my life I opened myself up to fully owning everything that came before, rather than having an experience and saying "get over it, Brooke! On to the next!" But in watching the film I was reminded that I'm very different now than I was as a kid. Different even than I was as a young adult in my twenties or thirties. I'm less fearful of the unknown. I don't have the rest of my life mapped out, like I thought I did back then—before I realized that any supposed "map" is more like a wish list. These days, I get a thrill from the awareness that my future is unknown. Anything can happen! I don't need to know what I want. I can figure that out as I go. What an adventure! I also feel fundamentally more grounded in this era of my life than I ever have (and not just because I know better than to get on a surfboard). I'm less focused on outside opinions, and I'm far less affected by criticism. I know I have done well, according to my own definition of success. All of this is a product of having been through every little moment highlighted in that film. And never has that success been more apparent than in the last scene of *Pretty Baby*, in which I sit down to dinner in my kitchen with my husband and daughters and discuss my career. The conversation was completely unplanned and was just supposed to provide some footage of us all together to be used during the credits. But in the scene, my girls began sharing thoughtful opinions and insight about my career and life. I was overcome with emotion listening to these smart, strong females. They have confidence! They can see things in my past that even I still struggle to see. These girls are their own women, and that is one of my proudest achievements. Throughout their upbringing I really tried to give them safe spaces to find out who they were independent of their mother. It's a lesson I think my mom resisted teaching me for fear I would abandon her. But I think it's *because* I give my daughters room to get to know and be themselves that they still want to connect with me. I guess, deep down, we always want our mommies. We crave being cared for. To feel safe. Even though I knew I was loved, I can't say I ever really felt safe. My girls do. And that makes me feel proud.

When I got that standing ovation at Sundance (now there's a phrase I never thought I'd get to write), I was nearly paralyzed with shock. There's something disarming about being applauded for enduring your life when it's the only life you've ever known. At first I didn't know how to take it, so I tried to hang back. But then Ali was standing behind me, literally shoving me to the front of the stage, forcing me to take in the celebration and accept the credit. And she didn't do that for my ego. It wasn't about making me feel like some superstar. She did it so that I could see that I deserve to feel proud of who I am and how I have lived. The applause was proof that I didn't let the world beat me down. The media who tried to spin my story or the journalists who tried to put me on the defensive or the men who tried to take my dignity—none of them succeeded. And boy did they try (and probably always will). They tried over and over to pull the rug out from under me, but I became Aladdin. Everyone who tried to take me down, I wouldn't let them, because frankly I didn't respect them enough to give them that much power.

In pushing me out in front of the crowd, Ali was reminding me of what I'm reminding you: It's okay to be applauded. And if no one else is clapping, then for god's sakes give yourself your own standing ovation. We can't keep handing over credit to others for our accomplishments, because they will keep taking it—and then some. Just getting to our fifties, living our lives, raising kids if we so choose—those are feats in and of themselves. Hopefully you had support along the way, but that doesn't mean you don't deserve to be acknowledged and celebrated for how you made it through. After all, you'd certainly be left with the blame if it had all gone horribly wrong.

It was surreal to look out at a roomful of people clapping for me and honoring my story. But I felt that they were applauding something else, too. The women in that room were clapping because they realized they weren't alone in their experiences and weren't crazy to feel the way they did. They could relate, in their own way, to how I was underestimated and judged. Sometimes you can only fully see your journey by witnessing someone else's, and I hope that's what the documentary did for the women who watched it. It was one woman's story, and a story that has played out in a very public and sometimes bizarre way, but what I felt in the applause was more about gratitude than praise. (Maybe I'm just struggling—still—with accepting any sort of praise . . . but I'll keep working on that with my therapist.) In that moment in the theater, which played out almost in slow motion, I felt that people were saying thank you, to me and to the whole documentary team, for showing them they're not alone. For empowering them to come to terms with their pasts—as complicated as they might be—so that they can have a happier future.

4

Bradley Cooper, Guardian Angel

GRAPPLING WITH THE END

Five days before my debut at The Carlyle, we put on an informal run-through for family and friends at a piano bar near my house. It was the first time I had done the show in its entirety in front of people, and I was quite nervous. I was scared mostly that something would go wrong with my voice, so I kept downing more and more water. Singing coaches have always urged the importance of staying hydrated, and I'm nothing if not an obedient student.

I was scheduled to fly to Indianapolis that afternoon to perform the show at a benefit concert. My director, Nate, and my pianist, Garret, came to my house after the run-through to wait for a car to the airport. Although I'd been doing everything I could to stay healthy for the Indy show, I was also stressed, which meant I wasn't sleeping well, and I didn't have a huge appetite. Still, I felt pretty good. And yet when Nate offered to get us coffees for the car ride, he looked at me as if something was off.

"Are you okay?" he asked as we walked to my front door. I'd decided to run to the pharmacy while Nate and Garret grabbed the coffees.

"Yeah, great," I said.

"You're sure?" he said. To hear Nate tell the story, I told him I was fine four times, but each time, he could see in my eyes that something wasn't right. My mouth was saying "I'm fine" while my eyes had that sort of dead Chucky stare you might use to try to telepathically communicate that "there's a creepy man behind me, I'm going to pretend everything's okay but please, send help." Except there was no creepy man behind me, and no matter how many times Nate asked, I insisted I was A-OK. I even gave him an emphatic two thumbs-up. Eventually he had to take me at my word (or hand gestures).

Nate and Garret went to get coffee, and I walked toward the pharmacy. But then I remembered I'd already been to the pharmacy that day—*wow, I really* was *out of it*—so I changed course and walked back toward my house, stopping in L'Artusi, the Italian restaurant near my place. Chris and I are regulars at L'Artusi (we even named our puppy, Tuzi, after it), and the sommelier had just sat through the run-through. I wanted to thank her.

I learned later that a friend of a friend, someone I'd been connected with over email but had never met, passed me on the street as I was walking from the pharmacy to the restaurant. She told our mutual friend that she had planned to approach me and introduce herself, but that I "looked agitated." The thing is, I never look agitated in public. I have certainly *been* agitated in public, but I've also been caught off guard by enough paparazzi to know how to keep the emotion off my face while I'm out and about. Clearly, something was off.

When I walked into L'Artusi, two women approached before I could make my way to the sommelier. I didn't know them, but they knew me. I'm used to that at this point. I think they had seen the documentary and wanted to discuss it, but the truth is I can't really remember what they said, because right at that moment, I just dropped. I went straight to the floor like a lead balloon, hitting my head on a table on my way down. Then, I started shaking, foaming at the mouth, and turning blue.

I was having a grand mal seizure.

I don't remember most of what happened during the episode—I've pieced it together largely from what other people have told me and what I saw on the L'Artusi security cameras. On the video, you can see me gesticulate while talking to the two fans, and then I start to gesticulate a bit more wildly, and then suddenly my hands drop and I go down. I would say it was terrifying, but the truth is that it was probably much scarier for the people who witnessed it.

I know now that one of the two ladies I was speaking with when I started to seize was a registered nurse (what luck!), so she made sure I was turned on my side while the folks at the restaurant called for help. I have a vague memory of hearing the word "tongue," but could that be the actress in me adding to the post-event script? Perhaps. I truly believe I heard it, but my husband says I'm being dramatic! (Not that he was even there.) Anyway, the next thing I remember, I'm opening my eyes on a gurney in an ambulance, with an oxygen mask on . . . and Bradley Cooper is sitting next to me, holding my hand in both of his.

Well, I guess I didn't make it, I thought to myself. *It was a good run.*

It turned out I was very much alive, and I really was being held by Bradley Cooper.

I should back up here to note that Bradley lives in our neighborhood and is a close friend of our family. His arrival at my side wasn't completely out of nowhere, though it definitely felt that way when I came to and saw his face in front of mine. What actually happened is that the hostess at L'Artusi called Chris, who was in the car on his way out to the beach. The hostess had also called my assistant, who contacted Bradley's assistant, who in turn called Bradley. When I opened my eyes, it was Bradley's bright blue eyes gazing back at me. "Brooke, I'm going with you to the hospital, okay?" he said. He'd brought two huge cops with him to caravan us to the hospital, sirens and all. Where he found these guys, I'll never know. I was very foggy but still silently laughed at the ridiculousness of it all. (They don't usually let nonrelatives ride in the ambulance with a patient, but I guess if American Sniper is with you, the rules don't apply.)

We arrived at the NYU emergency room a few minutes later. That's when I was informed that not only did I have a grand mal seizure but I also had peed my pants. (Fun fact: the only thing worse than peeing your pants is being told after the fact that you peed your pants while being held by Bradley Cooper.)

My seizure, I soon learned, was a result of low sodium levels. New York City was in the middle of a heat wave, and between drinking excessive amounts of water to prep for the show—three gallons during our run-through alone!—and sweating profusely due to the weather, I had flushed the sodium in my blood to dangerously low levels. Plus, I wasn't eating enough, because I was prepping for the show around the clock and had lost my appetite due to nerves, and food is another source of sodium. We're told to hydrate, hydrate, hydrate all our lives, but it turns out if you go overboard, it can be extremely dangerous! Who knew?!?

Chris soon arrived at the hospital, and he sat on the right side of the bed and Bradley on the left. My eyes kept switching from left to right, as if I were at a tennis match (I've been to a few in my lifetime). I still wasn't really able to talk, so I just kept nodding as Bradley emphatically told me I had to cancel Indianapolis and get strong for The Carlyle. Chris added that he would book me a flight to Indianapolis for the next day in case they released me and I could make the performance. (He had no intention of booking me a flight but he also knew I've never been one to cancel any performance, and this was the only way to get me to agree.)

I ended up in the hospital overnight. The whole experience was mortifying and devoid of any integrity. When I arrived, the nurses stripped me naked and wiped me down with some sort of baby wipe—I still don't really know what that was all about. Then they put in a catheter, which they had a lot of trouble inserting because I have a ton of scar tissue from a cone biopsy from decades ago (more on that in chapter 5 and I bet you can't wait . . .). Then, as if all that wasn't humbling enough, the nurses kept reminding me to shift my body from time to time so I didn't get bedsores. Nothing makes you feel young again like the threat of bedsores. The one blessing was that Bradley was not a witness to this particular portion of my ER stint.

It's easy for me to laugh off the whole episode now, but at the time, I was not amused. Scared, yes. Shocked, for sure. Angry? That, too. One of the most frustrating parts of the experience was the (male) doctors, who treated me like a silly little actress who didn't know what was good for her. "Have you been restricting your salt intake?" they asked condescendingly. "You really shouldn't limit your salt intake just to lose water weight!"

I wanted to slap them across the face with my peed-in pants! I responded with a curt, "Hey, excuse me"—ever the polite one—"I'm a fifty-eight-year-old woman. I actually look *younger* when I'm bloated. Eating salt is like Botox for me. So NO, I have not been limiting my salt intake to look skinnier or lose weight, thankyouverymuch!" This wasn't the result of some fad diet, and I certainly didn't appreciate the insinuation that I was a dumb celebrity who was sacrificing her health to look thin. I was singing more than I'd ever sung in my life, in a heat wave, while also hosting a podcast. I thought water would help me stay energized and keep my voice strong, because that's what they tell you. Until I ended up foaming at the mouth as if I were a fancy dish at the French Laundry.

The whole experience was terrifying, and the prescription ("eat more potato chips") didn't exactly meet the severity of the moment. But if you can believe it, this was only the second scariest health episode I'd had in the last few years.

The first came in January 2021. For the previous ten months, pretty much since the beginning of COVID, I'd been practicing standing on a balance board. For the uninitiated, a balance board is an oval wooden disc that looks like a small skateboard, but without wheels. It comes with a cylinder that sort of looks like a foam roller, and the idea is that you lay the roller on the floor, put the board on top, and then stand on it to balance. Conquering the balance board was one of my lockdown goals, and it took me a full year, but I did it. Once the world began to open up again, I returned to the gym and began using the balance board at the end of each workout as a method of centering myself and engaging my core. This particular day, I happened to be on the final workout of a ten-week physical challenge and was probably in the best shape of my adult life.

"You make it look so easy," this guy said to me one day after I hopped off the board. I didn't know him, but we were working out near each other, and he was just being friendly.

"It took me a while, but if you want to learn, you can," I said.

"I don't think so."

"Well, that's a defeatist attitude," I noted. "Here, let me show you." I got on the board, found my balance, and then I did the thing you're never supposed to do: I took my gaze off my spot, because I wanted to make sure that this man, who I didn't even know, was watching. Enter my ego! Almost immediately I lost my balance, flew in the air, and landed on my right hip with such force that I snapped my femur in half. Ambulances were called and paramedics arrived from two different locations. I was on the floor, and any attempt to sit up elicited primal guttural sounds that I'd never heard from myself, or from anybody else for that matter. It took multiple people, and I assume a good amount of morphine, to load me on the gurney paddle and position me vertically into the tiny elevator to exit the prewar building.

I was in the hospital for an entire month. First for surgery on my femur and the rehab and recovery from that, and then for a staph infection that developed in my arm at the site of my IV. That infection, which also resulted in a blood clot, was much scarier to me than the broken bone. Yes, the femur is the largest bone in your body, and breaking it is no small thing. I cannot adequately describe the excruciating pain except to say that I sounded like some mythical creature who was half woman, half dragon, possibly giving birth without drugs. But I kept thinking, *It's a bone. It will heal.* The staph infection is when I really got scared. At first the doctors didn't know if it was MRSA, which is the kind of infection that's resistant to antibiotics, and if it was, they said it could be life-threatening. After each test, I was waiting for results just *knowing* that I was about to be told that something was fatally wrong. It felt inevitable. And, because it was during COVID, I was all alone in the hospital—no visitors allowed—so everything felt even more fatalistic. It was just the state of the world at the time. It took a week to get the lab results because the specimen had to grow in the lab for them to be able to properly test it. Luckily, the infection wasn't MRSA, and antibiotics did the trick. But the fear, throughout that whole journey, was very real and incredibly isolating.

When you're in your midfifties, in the hospital for days or even weeks, you have no choice but to acknowledge your own mortality. You don't think about it much as a kid, or in your twenties or thirties, because time seems to stretch out before you.

You assume you've got forever. But there comes an age where dying is something you think about. Not constantly or daily, hopefully, and it's not that you are worrying or wondering how you're going to go. But there's an awareness, that wasn't always there, that time is finite. You've suffered losses, you've grieved, and you may even have had a few health scares yourself. If you're in the hospital for a broken femur, and you're surrounded by ninety-year-olds with broken hips . . . well, let me tell you, in that case you're *really* faced with the reality that the end comes for all of us. But even if not, at a certain age you start to see how fast the time goes, and how fleeting life can be. Having children only adds to that, in a "circle of life" kind of way, especially as your own parents age. I lost my parents a relatively long time ago—my dad died in 2003, my mother in 2012—but I've recently watched several of my friends go through this rite of passage. It's a strange time, because when it happens you feel orphaned, and almost like a kid again. Having what felt like two near-death experiences brought all that up for me again. Both instances made me miss my mommy and daddy. You want to be nurtured when something scary happens, because it doesn't actually *feel* like that much time has passed since you were being taken care of, and yet you still need to be the nurturer. At one point during the staph infection ordeal Rowan asked me if I was going to die. And, of course, I wondered the same thing myself, but I had to reassure her. I couldn't be parented, because I had to be the parent.

What's important to note is that as much as all this talk of mortality may seem like the dark side of aging, I'd argue it's not all depressing. In fact, it's the opposite. Just because you think about death occasionally or recognize its inevitability—it doesn't mean you're *close* to death. It means you appreciate life. You live more thoughtfully, more fully. You approach relationships with more gratitude. You use your body a bit more intentionally. For so long I felt invincible, and I beat up my body with dancing or exercise or diets (oh my!). Now I'm more interested in honoring this vessel that carries me around. I revere it a little bit more. I still want to look and feel my best, but it's for me this time. I want to take care of myself! If I don't, no one else will.

During both the femur situation and the seizure episode, what I knew for damn sure was that I had so much more living I wanted to do. I don't move through each day declaring myself #blessed, but I do recognize that I really like my life. And knowing that, and just how much I want to be here, makes this era a lot more meaningful than the decades when I spent so much time worrying or coveting things I didn't have such that I forgot to enjoy myself.

When I was in the hospital for a month with no visitors, I felt incredibly lonely. Though I haven't been a practicing Catholic in years, I remember thinking, *This is why people have religion.* When you have a belief system in place, you don't feel as alone, even in the scary moments, because you honestly believe that something, or someone, is looking out for you. You feel connected to something larger.

While I may no longer have the same faith that a guy with a beard in white robes and sandals is my savior, something did happen in that hospital room that made me believe angels are all around us. On a particularly hard day, during which I'd been told that my blood count was not improving and I'd have to stay even longer and have even more blood transfusions, a beautiful, dark-skinned, lean man, who aided the nursing staff, came into my room to empty the bedpan (not at all humiliating!). He saw my sad, tear-stained face and said, "Oh, it's a bit of a tough day is it?" I apologized and said I was fine, just a little sad. He then asked my permission to sing. I nodded, and this gentle man stood at the foot of my bed and sang a beautiful rendition of Michael Jackson's version of "Smile." His facial features were so refined and yet open and joyful. I cried even harder now, because there was gratitude and comfort mixed with the fear and sadness. His voice was stunning. He finished the song and said I had to believe that everything would be okay. I never saw him again, but the experience instilled in me a certain level of belief. Not in the dogma of organized religion but in the importance of human connection; in seeing and being seen. The interaction made me feel like I was no longer disappearing.

Connection was especially important for me during that long hospital stay because I didn't have the comfort of family around. (Not only could I not have visitors but my girls were too creeped out by my many cords and wires to want to FaceTime with any regularity.) I decided to make my situation feel more human by creating at least a small connection with every nurse or orderly I regularly interacted with. I needed to feel like a person and not just a number in a bed, which is what the health care system can feel like, especially if you're alone or can't advocate for yourself for whatever reason. I made a goal to remember one thing about each person who came into my room—the nurse who took my vitals had a two-year-old son whose birthday party was on Zoom, the guy who emptied my garbage can was thinking about proposing to his girlfriend, that sort of thing. Each time that person came through my space, we would talk. *Did your son like his present? Have you gone shopping for rings?* We had an honest exchange, and those conversations transformed the experience from one that felt isolating and scary to something a little less lonely.

It's not unlike what we all experienced in 2020. A global pandemic is an undeniable reminder that nothing in this life, and no amount of time, is a given. My family was on spring break in the

Bahamas when the world shut down. We had plans to be there for two weeks, but then we started to hear about schools closing and companies going remote. There was talk of restrictions around leaving the island, and questions regarding which boats would be allowed in and out, and we knew we didn't want to get stuck. We had been there only a few days when we booked a flight home, picked up the dog, packed up our things in Manhattan, and relocated outside the city. We ended up staying there for six months. Grier graduated eighth grade on Zoom; Rowan completed a year of high school that way. It was a scary and sad time for us for all the reasons it was scary for everyone—so many unknowns, so much loss. But on a more immediate level, in our nuclear family, I was one of those people who enjoyed being forced to slow down and spend time with my husband and kids. I understand how lucky I am to say that. How privileged I am that I could afford to forgo work, that I had a space to safely pass the months, that everyone in my family was healthy and would remain so. But when I could focus on what was in front of me, I had so much appreciation for this forced togetherness. I loved finding old-school ways to occupy our time. We played dominoes and did puzzles. We had a family Met Gala, just the four of us playing dress-up. The girls weren't on their phones constantly because none of their friends were going out and there was less to keep up with, so we cooked and went clamming and organized and exercised. And we appreciated it—or at least, I did—because we were together as we faced, every day, the fragility of it all.

When you experience any kind of health scare you're given a bit of a wake-up call, and I have a tendency to look for meaning in those moments. I always want to know what I'm meant to learn from a hard situation. If I can figure out *why* something bad happened, or what lesson I am supposed to take away from it, then maybe I can prevent it from happening again. But, of course, life doesn't work that way. As Chris reminds me any time I try to figure out the why, sometimes stuff just *is*. You fall down in a restaurant and wake up with Bradley Cooper holding your hand. You spend a year conquering the balance board, only to take a horrible tumble while teaching someone else. When I broke my femur, everyone around me wanted to find a reason. *Do you need to slow down? Are you out of balance? Was this the universe's way of giving you a break?* No, it's not. Sometimes shit just happens. It's hard to accept that, because it feels like chaos, but it's the truth. It doesn't mean you aren't thankful enough or that you're moving too fast or your priorities are out of whack. Sometimes there is no rhyme or reason.

When I was alone in the hospital, it was hard to know what to do with the knowledge that my accident wasn't about much other than me losing my balance, but I tried to make it a learning experience. And what I learned was something I think I would have gotten to eventually—I was heading there by virtue of my age. I learned that our time is short. That it's healthier, and so much more fun, to celebrate what you do have rather than what you don't. That every day is actually a gift. All those clichés? Turns out they're true!

These days, I smile and laugh at being able to go to my house and open the door and get kisses from my puppy and hugs from my family, and that I get to continue seeing how it all will unfold. I feel lucky for these real-life moments. They remind me that I don't need to look for the meaning behind the individual events of my life, because the meaning is right there in front of me—in my home and the people who inhabit it. It's a reminder that I want to live longer. I want more time. I want to have fun and see what else I can do. Did I need to bonk my head on a restaurant table in order to realize all this? Probably not. But it certainly made me look at this period of time and say, *Don't waste it. You still feel good and strong and alive, and you won't forever.* As much as I'll always choose humor and sarcasm over earnestness, I guess we're susceptible to these moments of sincerity as we age, too.

I read an incredible study[1] recently about this very quest for life's great meaning. It found that in our younger decades, like our twenties and thirties, we're more focused on figuring out what we're here for—and that constant existential searching has a negative correlation with mental health. It can cause stress and unhappiness. But as you enter your forties and fifties, and your life is more settled, the active search for meaning fades away while the perception that your life *already is meaningful* increases. At age sixty, the researchers said, "presence of meaning" peaks. In other words, at sixty years old—and in the immediate lead-up to it—we are more likely to feel our lives are meaningful just the way they are. Is there anything more hopeful?

And this isn't just about the spiritual or philosophical side of life. Presence of meaning is important to physical health and emotional well-being, according to this study. In a press release about the findings, Dilip Jeste, Distinguished Professor of Psychiatry and Neurosciences at UC San Diego School of Medicine, explained it this way: "Many think about the meaning and purpose in life from a philosophical perspective, but meaning in life is associated with better health, wellness and perhaps longevity. . . . When you find more meaning in life, you become more contented, whereas if you don't have purpose in life and are searching for it unsuccessfully, you will feel much more stressed-out."

For me, finding that meaning, and really enjoying my life, certainly has some connection to knowing that there will come an end.

Hopefully not anytime soon! But as I age, and become more aware that we don't have forever, I am more appreciative of my time and more eager to use it in ways that I enjoy. That's reason enough for me to take a dance class or eat another bowl of Häagen-Dazs, or say what I want to say without worrying constantly about what will happen or what others will think. It helps me appreciate the vividness of life, and live more firmly in the present.

I used to live in the wreckage of the future. In fact, I still need to frequently remind myself not to spiral into the what-ifs. There is absolutely no way I can predict what will happen, so why bother stressing when all I can do is be here now? It's taken a while, but I have many more days where I don't hunt for all the ways things might go wrong, and I just concentrate on what is actually happening in the moment.

Some days, I'll be walking down the street with my daughters and notice a full moon over the New York City skyline, or a beautiful sunset over the beach in Southampton, and I'll have one of *those moments*. You know the ones, when you're struck by the natural beauty of the world or overcome with emotion because we get to live in it. If you're anything like me, those thoughts are immediately followed by a question . . . *Am I drunk??? What's come over me?* If I try to pass this appreciation on to my kids, they roll their eyes and say, "Mom's getting sappy again! Everyone let's appreciate the moon!!" Okay, fine. That's their job as teenagers, I get it. But when I'm reminded of my own mortality—when I end up in the hospital or lose someone I love—I think of those moments looking at the moon in the city I love, with the family I adore. Or being able to participate in the activities that bring me joy. If my kids want to poke fun, that's fine. I'll just roll my eyes right back.

"You know what?" I say. "One day you'll understand."

5

No Longer the Punching Bag

A PLEA FOR SELF-ADVOCACY

L ying in a hospital bed with a broken femur, and then a staph infection, the only thing I knew with absolute certainty was that the best person to advocate for my care, and perhaps the *only* person to advocate for my care, would be me. If I had pain, I couldn't just quietly mention it and hope it would be taken seriously—I had to insist. If a doctor was going to conduct a procedure, I couldn't simply trust I would be informed of all the risks or possible side effects or even what exactly was going to happen in the surgery—I had to ask. One of the benefits of age is learning from experience, and what I knew at fifty-seven, but not yet at twenty-seven, or even thirty-seven, was that although I hadn't gone to medical school, I knew my body best, and I was entitled to all the information regarding its care. Rather than blindly deferring to those who supposedly knew better, I had to be my own greatest champion.

For some reason, I never hesitated to voice my opinions at work. I've always felt comfortable sharing my ideas about what works in a script (especially when it comes to dialing up the humor) or what looks might work on a photo set. In my press interactions, I've tried to stand up for my convictions, from those pressure-filled interviews as a kid to Cruise-gate decades later. In so much of my life, this belief that I had important opinions came easily. But when it comes to advocating for my physical health, I've hesitated. Advocating for myself is something I've had to learn the hard way, a couple of times over.

In my midthirties, I had an irregular Pap smear, which required me to get a cone biopsy, which is a procedure to remove abnormal tissue from the cervix. It was a necessary procedure—the biopsy did in fact find abnormal cells in my cervical tissue, and those cells were categorized as CIN III, which meant they were severely abnormal and would have quite likely developed into cancer. When the procedure was over, the doctor gave me the good news: the biopsy was successful. They had to be aggressive with what they removed—they took out practically my entire cervix—but they got all the precancerous cells, with clear margins, and I was precancer free. This was indeed great news and a huge relief. Of course it was. But it was also the only news I was given. No one bothered to tell me, for example, that I'd been packed with gauze to stop the bleeding, and that the gauze would eventually fall out, and that this was normal. When that gauze suddenly fell out . . . well, I am not exaggerating when I tell you I thought I was hemorrhaging and dying, or else giving birth to something I didn't even know I was carrying. I felt like my entire uterus had fallen out onto the bathroom floor. The doctor also failed to mention that such an aggressive biopsy could result in so much scar tissue that it could become difficult to conceive. I didn't learn that little tidbit until years later. Chris and I hadn't exactly been *trying* to get pregnant, but we also weren't *not* trying. For two years, even before we were married, Chris and I operated under the agreement that if I got pregnant, so be it. We knew we wanted to get married and have a family, and if I was a bride with a baby bump, well, I'd just get my dress altered. But that was never necessary, and shortly after we got married

I went to the doctor to get checked out. She did an exam, and lo and behold, the scar tissue from the cone biopsy had tightened and shortened my cervix, which made it especially difficult to conceive. In fact, during my first round of IVF, there was so much scar tissue in my cervix that rather than passing a catheter through my cervical canal to my uterine cavity, the doctors had to go through my belly button to implant the embryo. I joked that because they went through my belly button, I could argue that I was still a virgin!

Amazingly, that first IVF round was successful, and I became pregnant—only to miscarry three months later. Because it was my first pregnancy, and I'd been so focused on the *getting* pregnant part, I'd never even thought about the possibility of *losing* the pregnancy. And then, in December 2001, I was backstage at MuppetFest, a fundraiser for Save the Children and a tribute to Jim Henson, when I got a call on my cell phone. At the time, I was standing under a towering Mr. Snuffleupagus while we both waited in the wings to go onstage. Earlier that morning I'd gotten some bloodwork for my still-very-early pregnancy, so when my phone rang, I was eager to pick it up. "I'm sorry," the voice on the line told me, "but the pregnancy is no longer viable." I looked up from my phone and saw Snuffy's big eyelashes blink at me, as if to say: "I'm sorry, little girl, but you'll be okay." (This moment is the opening scene of *Down Came the Rain*, and though it happened more than twenty years ago now, I still remember every detail.)

I was told I'd need to get a shot of methotrexate, a drug that would speed up my inevitable miscarriage, and what ensued was probably the worst twelve straight hours of my life. The thing about a miscarriage is—you have no choice but to just go through it. There's no cold compress that can make you feel better, nothing that can make the hours of pain pass more quickly. And unlike the pain of childbirth, there is no baby waiting for you on the other end. I spent that evening lying in my bed with my dog Darla at my feet—she would army crawl up to the pillow to lick my face and then go back down. I wouldn't let Chris in the room. The whole experience just felt like something I wanted to endure alone. Plus, I was so angry. It had been so difficult to get pregnant and I had wanted it for so long, and now I'd *almost* had it but lost it? I was pissed.

At some point, I took something to help me sleep. When I awoke about four or five hours later, the physical pain had subsided. I remember looking out the window that morning, mad at the entire world, and thinking to myself, *You are no longer a child. You have experienced something that took your innocence away.*

The miscarriage was so violent and excruciatingly painful that when it came time for a second IVF attempt I asked my doctor: "Do you think it hurt so much because the scar tissue was getting stretched? Is that possible??" She was willing to find out, and so my doctor attempted to access my uterine cavity with a catheter through my cervix, and for the first time, she was successful. "I'm in! I'm in!" she yelped, and I will never forget Chris looking up at her and deadpanning, "I say the same thing every time I'm down there."

It was my female fertility specialist who told me that my difficulty getting pregnant was probably a result of the cone biopsy. But the first doctor, the male who performed the biopsy, should have been the one to tell me. He shirked his duty as a medical professional, in my opinion. Would I have *not* gotten the biopsy if I'd known? Of course not. As I said, I almost certainly would have ended up with cancer if I hadn't gotten those cells removed. But I would have appreciated having the details so that I could have given *informed* consent. Had I been aware of the risks, I could have made other choices to support my fertility. Perhaps I would have been able to get the scar tissue attended to right away. Perhaps I would have gone to a fertility specialist earlier, to learn if the biopsy affected my ability to get pregnant, rather than spending two years secretly hoping, every month, that this would be the moment, only to be disappointed over and over. I spent a lot of time trying and wondering and beating myself up unnecessarily, feeling like a failure. Not to mention that six rounds of IVF costs a small fortune! I am quite aware of how lucky I was to be able to afford it.

I guess one could argue that I never asked the doctor how the biopsy could affect a potential pregnancy, but that seems a bit unfair. First, we don't ask what we don't know to ask, and when I was thirty-five, there was so much I didn't know to ask. I think I was actually more hesitant than the average person when it came to discussing bodily issues. Remember, my body was long the subject of public fascination, and my virginity made national headlines in the 1980s.

Second, I sincerely believed that most people knew better than I did. If a doctor said I needed something, who was I to question that recommendation? They would tell me what I needed to know. But I look back on that experience now and, I'll admit, it doesn't surprise me that it was a male doctor. I really believe that a woman probably would have said, "The margins are clear and that's great news, but just for the future, you should be prepared that this could affect your ability to get pregnant." It could have been as simple as that. Leaving that disclaimer out of our discussion seems wholly irresponsible, but I often wonder if that's just not on a male doctor's radar because it's not their anatomy. I imagine that if a man performed an operation that would affect his male patient's sperm count, he'd mention it. And yes, of course this is a generalization and there are plenty of wonderful male doctors who would have given me the information I needed, but this one certainly did not, and I spent countless hours wondering why my lifelong dream of becoming a mother was proving so difficult. I cried to a close girlfriend, saying, "Why can't I be normal? Maybe I've been given too much in life so I don't deserve this!" Every time I had my blood drawn only to be told "nope, sorry, try again next month" I felt completely hopeless.

About eight years later, after I'd had both my girls, I found myself in another—and in retrospect, much more egregious—situation where it felt like my medical care was taken out of my hands. I was at an appointment with my gynecologist, and after my exam she asked if I ever felt discomfort because of my labia.

"Only in tight jeans and spin classes and every romantic moment ever," I said.

(I do apologize if this is too graphic or simply TMI, as some generations still call it. I'd be lying if I said I'm not embarrassed to share this very intimate information. But, if we are to change the way we approach and talk about women's health, then we need to bring up the uncomfortable but very real issues. Shame is no longer an option. So, I'll go first.)

My labia (you've got to admit this is a funny word) had been an issue for me since I was in high school, and one I'd been ashamed of forever. My best friend Lisa had the same situation, and at least together we could laugh about it. It's like you're in a boxing gym and you have two little speed bags between your legs, we'd joke. It hurt and it was in the way, and when I told my gynecologist as much, she said it was very common and that I was surely a candidate for a labial reduction procedure. Technically it would be considered a cosmetic procedure—even that still pisses me off because we're talking about pain—but it was one that would significantly decrease my discomfort. Why should that be reduced to a cosmetic choice, as if I wanted a more photogenic labia so I could be in adult films (nothing against those in the profession!)? Labeling it (or labialing it? sorry!) "cosmetic" was not only unjust but it also meant that, like many other important procedures and treatments for women, it would not be covered by insurance. That could be the subject of a whole other book! In any case, my doctor made me feel less ashamed and relieved that there was a solution. She recommended a doctor in L.A. who was supposedly the best.

I had one consultation with this (yes, male) doctor and wondered why I hadn't heard about this surgery earlier—years of discomfort, potentially fixed! What a revelation! I made an appointment and went in not long after to have the procedure. When it was over, the doctor gave me the rundown of how it went, as they do. "I was very detailed," he said, to my relief and excitement. And then: "I was in there for four hours, and you know what I did? I tightened you up a little bit! Gave you a little rejuvenation!" He looked at me expectantly.

Wait, what?? I was shocked, speechless. I can't remember how I responded, or even if I said anything, but if I did, I think it was something as eloquent as "Oh?" Was I supposed to say thank you?

"After two kids, everything is looser," he said. But I had C-sections, and a scarred, more restricted cervix, I responded. "Still . . ." he said, staring, as if waiting for some further reaction from the lady whose feet were glamorously in the metal stirrups. He acted as if he'd done me a favor, and that I should, in fact, be grateful. There was a real "I threw this in for free, little lady" vibe to his delivery. But I had never asked to be "tightened" or "rejuvenated" (translation: given a younger vagina). It was not something I wanted. I felt numb. I got dressed, went to my car, and drove home in a stupor.

I was horrified, but also at a loss. I didn't want to sue this man—or maybe I did *want* to, but I didn't feel I could—because

I didn't particularly want talk of my lady parts, once again, on the front page of every paper. And yet . . . it was deeply upsetting. This man surgically altered my body without my consent. And he thought he had done me a *favor* by throwing in a "bonus procedure"? The sheer gall of it enraged me. The fact that the most intimate parts of my body had been a public focal point for so long . . . it was enough already. All I could think was, *Why can't everybody just leave my vagina alone?* (Even now, as I write this, I know this will be the bit that makes headlines. Whatever. Women deserve all the information.)

Had I been happy with the results of the procedure, I still would have been angry that he did it without my consent. But as it turns out, I wasn't happy with the results, and haven't been since. I can't be bothered to change anything now, but once I was healed, I definitely noticed a difference in my body, and not a good one. Maybe if I was someone who was obsessed with sex I'd have been happy for the "freebie," but I'd say my sex drive is pretty typical for a woman my age. I like intimacy, but I don't need it every day. And the truth is, the procedure did not enhance my pleasure. Maybe it was, in fact, a gift to my husband? And one even he did not ask for.

I never took action against this doctor. I never even spoke to him about it again, in part because I had started to question myself, to wonder if he was right, that I *should* feel lucky. Or maybe, I thought, this was a needed improvement for my man, who was secretly dissatisfied but would have never dared address the subject of my "loose down theres"? It's crazy to me that these ideas even popped into my head. What's even crazier is that I didn't even discuss it with my husband until later. I can't remember why I eventually told him, but he was nearly as angry as I was.

I moved to New York City shortly afterward and started filming *Lipstick Jungle* and pushed it out of my mind . . . until recently.

Because if the same thing happened today, my reaction wouldn't be so generous. Now when I think about that incident, it's not tinged with shame or guilt or any sort of wondering if maybe I should be thankful. My sentiment is basically a giant middle finger. Fuck that guy! He had no right to do what he did, and if it happened to me now, I would make my own blaring headline and blast it everywhere. That's what this age feels like to me, and I like it so much better.

For years I accepted as fact that doctors knew best, but now my first instinct is: "I know myself better than you do. I've lived in this body for almost sixty years. You may be a professional and have plenty of medical expertise, but I know my body." And again, this is not a referendum against all male doctors—I've had some great ones—but I struggle to believe it's a coincidence that both of these really disorienting medical episodes (not to mention the interrogation about my salt intake after my seizure) occurred with men.

Receiving an unsolicited vaginal rejuvenation can't really be chalked up to a lack of self-advocacy. I could have asked all the right questions and explained exactly what I wanted, and unless I'd known to say "please do not 'tighten me up,' even if you think you're doing me a favor," I couldn't have gotten ahead of this. But by the time the broken femur came around, I had come to realize that I needed to be vocal about my medical care. I had to ask questions and be clear about what I wanted and needed, and also what I didn't want or need. I knew that if the doctors tried to dismiss me, I simply had to ask again, and if that didn't work, speak louder.

The ability to self-advocate is not exactly a factor of age but of experience, though of course those pieces are related. I saw an article recently titled "The Art of Being a Difficult (aka Empowered)

Patient," and that headline got right to the issue. As girls, we're taught to be polite, to comply, to defer. At least, that's what was drilled into me from a young age. If we don't, we're "difficult." I've always tried to teach my girls the opposite lesson. But even if you're raised with an emphasis on compliance, there comes a certain age when the desire to be liked stops taking priority. I'm not always one to use phrases like "step into your power," but I do think that's what happens at this age, and especially with regard to self-protection. We're at our personal nexus of self-knowledge and confidence and fortitude, and that manifests in our ability to speak up and fight for ourselves and those we love. It's not that we're angry, but we're also done walking on eggshells so that nobody, God forbid, *thinks* we're angry.

And research shows that age really does play a factor when it comes to medical self-advocacy in female patients. A study published in the journal *Advances in Nursing Science* found that "compared to younger individuals, older individuals report higher levels of engagement in decision-making and effective communication, perhaps due to having more experiences with the health care system in general."[1] This study specifically looked at female cancer patients but notes that self-advocacy is "imperative in all health care settings." The more you are required to care for your health, the better you get at doing it.

All this proved pivotal when I broke my femur, because after I was taken from the gym where I fell to the ER, I was immediately taken to surgery. Unbeknownst to me, I was supposed to only be stabilized in the ER and then transferred to the Hospital for Special Surgery, where a specialist was scheduled to operate the following day. But the doctor on call at the ER, who was not a femur specialist but an ankle guy, took it upon himself to do the surgery right away. Did he not know he was supposed to wait? Was he trying to be a hero? Did he think he could figure it out like he would an ankle? I don't know. I was not conscious for any of these decisions. The surgeon put a metal rod into my hip, and another one down the length of my femur. But, by mistake, he neglected to secure the plate *or* the broken bone in place. When I woke up, everything looked great and the discomfort had dissipated significantly, but within a few hours, an excruciating pain hit, as if the break had happened all over again. I was howling in agony, and I knew something was wrong, but the doctors and nurses weren't convinced. They assumed that since I was just coming out of the anesthesia, the pain was creeping back in. Deferred pain, one doctor called it. Well, I wanted to defer pain to this guy's balls! Something was very wrong, and they were talking to me like I was just some hysterical female. Which as an actress I could have easily obliged simply to get another goddamned X-ray. And listen. I do have a high pain tolerance. Always have. But there's pain, and then there's *pain*, and this was the latter. I begged them to give me another X-ray.

"We X-rayed you after the surgery," the doctor said.

"I know," I said. "But I'm telling you. I'm in real pain here. Do me a favor and X-ray it again. I'll pay for it if that's the issue." I couldn't figure out why this had become such a battle when there was no question, as far as I could tell, that something was wrong. But research shows that this is how it often is for women in pain. Study after study has found a gender bias in the medical field that results in women's suffering not being taken seriously, and thus not relieved. A 2021 study published in the *Journal of Pain* found that when both genders express the same amount of pain (via their facial expressions), women's discomfort is considered less intense.[2] "If the stereotype is to think women are more expressive than men, perhaps 'overly' expressive, then the tendency will be to discount women's pain behaviors," coauthor Elizabeth Losin said in the study's press release. "The flip side of this stereotype is that men are perceived to be stoic, so when a man makes an intense pain facial expression, you think, 'Oh my, he must be dying!'" I had to laugh when I read this, considering how often my girlfriends and I commiserate over how our husbands fall apart at the first sign of a cold while we're expected to always, *always*, power through and continue to care for everyone around us.

Other studies have found that women with chest pain waited nearly 30 percent longer than men to be seen by a doctor and evaluated for a possible heart attack;[3] that women with chest pain are twice as likely as men to be diagnosed with mental illness;[4] that women with acute abdominal pain were 25 percent less likely to be given opioid painkillers.[5] And it's worse for women of color, whose pain is treated with even less seriousness. A 2019 study found that Black patients are 40 percent less likely than white patients to be given medication for acute pain.[6] Another study found that a "substantial number" of white medical students and residents believed white and Black patients experienced pain differently.[7] "False beliefs about biological differences between blacks and whites continue to shape the way we perceive and treat black people—they are associated with racial disparities in pain assessment and treatment recommendations," the study's authors write. Black women sit at this intersection, which means their pain is underestimated twice over.

While I'm certain I was experiencing the same discounting that many women face, I have to recognize that I'm one of the lucky ones. I'm famous, and with fame comes power. Doctors are probably more inclined to pay attention to me as a result, or to take precautions they wouldn't otherwise. They don't want it to be known that they made a mistake on a famous person. Perhaps they were quicker to indulge my insistence on an X-ray because I am Brooke Shields. That's an uncomfortable reality for me and shameful of them, but I admit that it helps me get what I need sometimes. Though my pain is by no means more important than the next woman's, it will often get tended to more quickly. But there's a flip side, which I have also experienced—sometimes being a public figure is a liability. People will deliberately ignore me to prove that they don't care that I'm me and because they assume that I will want some kind of special attention. Or they become enamored and lose sight of the matter at hand. In college, teachers were always worried that others might think they were being lenient with me, and as a result they were harder on me. When it comes to medical situations, because I am not only famous but also a famous *woman*, there seems to be a default assumption that I will be bitchy and demanding. A diva. As a result, I have to kill doctors with kindness—I mean, really overdo it—just to prove that I'm a human who doesn't want *extra* attention, but does want to be treated fairly. Eventually I was brought in for a second X-ray and, what do you know, it turned out that the broken part of the bone had popped off the metal rod and was jutting out. My pain was not a figment of my imagination but a symptom of a surgery gone wrong.

So I got a second surgery, with a new doctor, in which they put in more rods and a metal plate. But first, I had to essentially fire the ankle specialist. I wanted to be enraged. He should have had the humility to say "maybe a femur guy is better equipped to operate here." But also, he was the ER doctor on call when I arrived at the hospital. He'd probably been instructed to stabilize me, which might be what he thought he was doing. I couldn't know for sure, and although he didn't apologize in the least (that would be admitting a mistake) or even seem sorry, I didn't want to publicly shame him for doing what he thought was right. Enter the femur specialist from HSS. He was an elegant, commanding man with thick gray hair and a South African accent who towered over the other surgeons and nurses in the room. As he walked to my bed, it was as if the seas had parted for Moses. He offered to operate on me the following day, in his OR if I so chose. Oh, I chose! But when I looked at ankle man, who I think had hoped I'd let him fix his mistake, I kind of felt bad for him. "These things happen!" I assured him. "But I'm going to go with this new plan." I was listening to myself and thinking, *Are you really this generous of a human, Brooke? Or are you just pathetic? Or have women truly been trained to make others feel better, even when we're the ones suffering?*

After surgery number two there was still a lot of pain, but it was the normal pain of a serious surgery and a tough recovery. I have to imagine the doctors would have found the problem eventually, but to be doubted and questioned and dismissed was a bit of a mind fuck. Luckily, I knew my body well enough to keep speaking up.

The staph infection that followed unfolded similarly. The same needle had been in my arm for days, even staying in place while I was transferred from one hospital to another. I kept saying, "You know, this is getting a little itchy. It seems kind of inflamed?" I know things itch when they heal, but I hadn't been injured in my arm, so there wasn't anything I should be healing *from.* Still, when I told the doctors about my concerns, I was told that "we don't want to keep poking and prodding you, so we'll leave it where it is." I eventually made friends with a night nurse who I convinced to take the needle out of my arm and put my IV somewhere else, but by then the damage was done. I went home shortly thereafter, only to wake up that first morning in my bed with an arm that looked like Popeye's. Back to the hospital I went!

Now I needed to get *another* surgery—this one to excavate and biopsy the tissue around the wound. I was getting prepped by an arrogant anesthesiologist, one who had also been in my previous femur surgery, about two weeks earlier.

"Remember me?" he asked as he pulled down his mask to show me his face. "You sure have had a go of it lately!"

I didn't want to be whiny or self-pitying, so I smiled and said, "Well, I've got good things in my life, and these are just little roadblocks."

Well, this mofo scoffs at me and, while tsking, says: "Trust me, when God was handing out good luck, you got your fair share!"

I was stunned. He left the room then came back to roll me to surgery. I could not let this one go! Who the hell did he think he was to cast judgment on me or my life? This man didn't know me. Clearly he *thought* he did, but he most certainly did not. I immediately cast my own judgment: he was obviously either a frustrated actor at heart or an anesthesiologist who felt he didn't get the proper respect for being a medical doctor. I felt a bit bitchy, but hey, I was the one about to go under the knife. And wasn't part of his job to help make me more comfortable and less fearful? I am not a doctor of any kind, but I assume that blatantly insulting the patient isn't in any medical book.

Still, how was I going to put him in his place before going into induced la-la land? I had to think fast. As we were rolling along to the operating room I said: "You know, something you just said back there has stuck in my craw." (I'd never used that phrase before, but it felt appropriately sarcastic in the moment.) Then I started to recount my whole history: born a tiny preemie two months early, divorced parents by five months of age, single mother with alcoholism, public scrutiny, loss, illness, kidnap threats, stalkers . . . I went on and on, listing everything I've had to endure or overcome. Then I stopped and ended calmly with: "Yeah, so I guess you and I have different definitions of luck."

He didn't say a word, then proceeded to try to find a vein,

which wasn't proving easy. I should have stopped there and shut up, but I was on a roll. If I was going to go out, I was going to do so fighting! "Can't find a vein, can you?"

"Well, where do you think I should put it!?" he asked.

"I went to Princeton, not anesthesiology school."

"Oh, well, here's one in your neck," he said.

"Oh good, so I can audition for Bride of Frankenstein."

"Just bear down," he said.

"Am I having a baby?"

He scoffed. Again.

"I do have one last thing to add before you put me under," I said. "I'm surprised you don't walk with a limp."

"What?"

I finished with: "It just must be so hard to walk straight with that huge chip on your shoulder."

The last thing I remember is seeing the eyes of all three nurses widen behind their masks, and their shoulders bouncing up and down with stifled laughter. I never even got to count backward.

That exchange was emblematic of the hospital stay that followed: I was going to have to be my own best friend. I would ask for extra physical therapy and rehab. I would listen, all day long, as doctors would confer within my earshot or talk to the nurses. I paid attention to what was being said about my care. Eventually I'd gathered enough knowledge about my situation that I could ask informed questions. I'd overhear a conversation and jump in and ask, "Oh, if you're saying *that* does it mean you'll have to do *this*?" One of those times, the doctors and specialists and interns were gathered around my bed, discussing my body, when I interjected with a question regarding antibiotics and white blood cells. Before responding to my very valid question, the infectious disease specialist turned to me with his most patronizing smile and tilt of his head, and answered my question with a question of his own: "Have you been browsing WebMD?" I wanted to scratch his eyes out. Instead I replied, "No, if I'd been on WebMD I'd be convinced you are all trying to kill me. I've actually been listening and paying attention while you've been speaking about me as if I'm not present, or just can't hear you." I was on a roll! The room went silent, and I just stared at him waiting for an answer. I was pleasant and even kept a wee smile on my face.

"Well, Miss Shields" (I'm not sure if he intended to say "miss," but I took it as a compliment), "that's actually a good question, and yes, there could very well be a correlation between the two." No shit! God, I hate being condescended to!

That doctor's insulting WebMD question is probably why I got so ticked off when the seizure doc asked if I'd been restricting my salt. This assumption that I couldn't possibly know how to do anything, including how to take care of myself, was infuriating—not to mention that his question implied that I'd somehow caused my own seizure. I know these doctors would never say they were victim blaming, but would it have hurt them to give me the benefit of the doubt? To talk to me with the assumption that I was smart, rather than defaulting to the assumption that since I was pretty, or female, or in my fifties, I must not know anything?

I'm not a health care expert. Not even close. But I am a Brooke Shields expert. We each are the experts of our own experiences. And yet as women we are not always encouraged to familiarize ourselves with our own bodies. Even in pregnancy, I went to the doctor once a week but rarely was I actually asked how I was feeling. My OB would check that everything was in order with the baby, and then send me on my way. And now that my baby-making days are behind me? Well, to hear some doctors tell it, all that's left of me is hot flashes and menopause. I'm a ball of fire, and a diminishing one at that.

Obviously, I know different. If you've ever experienced something similar—and if you're a woman of a certain age, you probably have—well, you know different, too.

If getting older comes with an increased awareness of our mortality, that's accompanied by an increased appreciation for our physical health. Nothing is a given when you've seen loss or suffered health scares, so I pay close attention these days. If something feels off, I flag it, no matter how bothersome or overly curious I might come off to the doctor or specialist. I'm much more forward about asking that any tests or procedures be made clearer to me prior to moving forward, because it's my right and responsibility. If a doctor wants to write me off due to my gender or my age, I can't stop them, but that doesn't mean I'll defer to them or shrink to accommodate their assumptions. I'm not going to shy away from advocating for myself to make someone else more comfortable, and that's exactly what I tell my daughters, what I hope they learn now so that they can get a head start: don't be afraid to ask questions. There is information available, but the only way to get it is to ask. The only way to ensure your desires or concerns are taken seriously is to voice them. As loud as is necessary.

I fight for myself because I can, and because I have to. I do not want to wake up to another "Surprise! Guess what I did for you?" from any doctor, ever. If it sounds like self-advocacy takes a lot of effort, well, that's because it does. Aging is empowering, but it isn't always easy. It takes resilience. Luckily, by now we have that in spades.

6

More Than Just a Pretty Face

WE CONTAIN MULTITUDES

Not long ago, I was walking down the street and passed a group of four teenage girls—or maybe they were in their early twenties—taking a bunch of selfies. They were posing and positioning themselves for their best angles, and I heard one of them say to another, "Okay, that looks good, I just don't want any of my fat to show."

I still can't believe I did this, but I guess the mom in me took over because I spun on my heels and marched right up to them. "You don't know me," I said, "but I'm a mother and my daughters are around your age and I couldn't help overhearing what you were saying and I just have to tell you: you are all beautiful and you have to stop doing this to yourselves, and the sooner the better. You are young and stunning and different and interesting, and it's a lifetime of pain if you can't stop picking yourselves apart."

One lesson that decades of being photographed has taught me is that so many of the things we bemoan about our bodies are hardly unique to us—they're features everyone has, they're just airbrushed out of the photos we see in magazine covers or on movie posters. No matter who you are, you're not the only person with cellulite or blemishes or armpit skin that sticks out a bit when you wear a tank top. And yet, we are convinced that these supposed "flaws" are the most important things about us, and we become obsessed with "fixing" them.

I am certainly not immune to this urge to fixate on my least-favorite parts. For example, these days when I look down at my knees and thighs it's as if Silly Putty has melted into a frown around my kneecaps. When I have a movie to promote or a modeling job on the horizon, I've found myself taping my thighs to my Spanx—literally pulling my skin up from my knees and adhering it to my shapewear for an immediate (and surgery-free!) lift. (I learned this trick from using kinesiology tape on my knees to dance in Broadway shows.) But when I see young girls berating themselves for looking anything less than 100 percent perfect from all angles, it tears me up inside. I am well aware that the skin of my thighs has nothing to do with my value as a human, but I'm not sure these girls feel the same way. They think their physical appearance is some sort of commentary on who they are, and that breaks my heart.

Of course, one reason why these girls—all girls—are so hard on themselves is that unrealistic beauty standards have become the cultural norm. I can't deny that I played a role in contributing to those standards. I was in those skintight Calvins. I was on the cover of *Life* in 1983 in an itty-bitty red bathing suit next to the headline: BROOKE BRINGS BACK THE BIKINI. I don't regret doing those jobs, because they paid the bills and afforded me the life I lived, but I can look back and see that I helped perpetuate certain myths about how women should look. I'm not sure this matters, but I can say with complete honesty that I didn't realize those implications at the time. First of all, because I was young, and in many ways a victim of the same beauty standards that I helped establish. But also because we weren't having conversations like this back then. All I knew was that my job was to look "good"—meaning to stay a certain size and maintain a pretty face—and I always wanted to do my job well. And sometimes that is still true. I still model, and I would be lying if I pretended I don't go into those jobs wanting to appear sexy and beautiful. That's what everyone wants me to be. And I want it, too. It feels good to photograph in a way that makes everyone happy. And I do believe that when I feel good about how I look, I feel better overall. But over the years I have also tried to use the platform my popularity afforded me—and still affords me—to contribute to this body-image conversation in positive ways. Still, I know that I can't decry today's beauty standards—which I do think have gotten more extreme with social media and the drastic increase in plastic surgery for young people—without acknowledging my contribution to them.

The ladies I bombarded on the street happily received my motherly advice until one of them did a double take and said, "Wait . . . aren't you . . . ?" and I said "yes" and the spell was broken. But they didn't ask for a selfie, and before I walked away I offered one last piece of unsolicited advice: "Listen, I understand the desire to photograph yourself from what you believe are your best angles. I do the same thing. But please find what you like about yourself and focus on that. Look for the qualities you can celebrate instead of fixating on the things you don't like. I'm trying to do you a favor—I want to save you years of agony!"

The noise of self-criticism begins when we're so young—around age twelve for girls, the author of *Confidence Code*, Katty Kay, pointed out. While age hasn't eliminated this chatter for me entirely, it has at least turned down the volume. That seems to be true for most women—as we age, we tend to be a little less hard on ourselves. I look at what my body has done for me—bearing and nourishing children, surviving trauma, healing from harm—and I have such appreciation for it. The entirety of what my body is capable of makes me proud, and recognizing its wisdom and resilience allows me to see it beyond the limitations of body image. But that's a perspective that comes with age. And experience. When we're young, society tells us to invest so much energy into how we look—and to derive our value from how others see us. As we mature, we can reflect and marvel at what our bodies have done for us, and that takes some of the onus off appearance as *the thing* that matters most.

The research bears this out. An AARP survey found that "52 percent of boomer women say that they are kinder to themselves about body image as they age, compared with 41 percent of Gen Xers and 38 percent of millennials."[1] I was born in the earliest years of Gen X, so it's nice to know that I can look forward to even more gentle internal messaging as I age. That same study found that 61 percent of women surveyed agreed with the statement "I am beautiful at any age." As we get older, I think a word like "beauty" takes on a deeper meaning. You might genuinely love everything about your appearance, but even if you don't, being beautiful becomes about more than just how you look in a photo or adhering to someone else's standards for what you should look like. You grow an appreciation for all of the nuances and idiosyncrasies, inside and out, that make you *you*.

I'm sure many of you have had conversations with the young women in your lives similar to the one I had with those girls on the street. We see their self-critical behavior, and it feels upsetting because we know it so well. We've lived with it for decades, and we may always live with it on some level. While I've come to appreciate my body, it would be a lie to say that I hit forty or fifty or fifty-five and overnight fell in love with everything about my appearance. In fact, I have never fully loved everything about my appearance.

I was labeled "beautiful" at an early age, which of course was nice to hear, but it wasn't something I was particularly proud of. My face was anointed, and it opened doors for me, and helped me earn a living. But my face wasn't something I achieved, it was something I was born with. Despite all the external validation, I've spent as much time as anyone else picking apart my appearance, or wishing I looked different or was thinner or, depending on the moment, wishing that I looked more like what I thought I was "supposed" to look like. (As often as my face was celebrated, I also lost jobs because I was not "all-American-looking.") I haven't always seen what others saw in my face or body, and I have wasted countless hours wishing I was more this, or less that.

People will often say to me, "But you were a supermodel!" However, that's not actually true. I was never a supermodel, because I never had that body. I was very specifically told I *was not* runway worthy, because I wasn't skinny enough. (In an industry where the only acceptable size was a sample size—that's a twenty-four-inch waist—I was the girl being sewn into dresses from behind because the clothes wouldn't zip.) Being told you are "the face," you begin to believe that's all you are—a face. That you don't have the right body. From the neck up, I was Brooke Shields, but it was like my body existed in a different reality. That feeling stays with you, no matter who you are. I was ashamed, because I felt like I was disappointing people. And the times when my body *was* the center of attention, it was commoditized and speculated upon in such a way that it didn't really feel like it belonged to me.

In 1981, I was interviewed by Barbara Walters in the wake of the Calvin Klein ads, and she asked me, on national television, what my measurements were. I was fifteen years old. And my mother was sitting right next to me! Even at the time I knew it wasn't right, but I behaved like a polite young woman and answered the question, because that's what I always did. Then Barbara asked me to stand up next to her, so we could compare our sizes. In the clip, I laugh awkwardly, because what other choice did I have? By then, incidents like that happened so often that I'd become comfortable in the discomfort. I actually stood up next to this very grown woman and let her compare our sizes. I felt taken advantage of, but I was so used to it that I became disassociated from my *self*. My body was public domain.

In reality, while I wish I could say that being on magazine covers boosted my confidence, the opposite was true. The more my looks were equated with my value, the harder I was on myself—not unlike those girls on the street. When I professed my insecurities to my first husband, he would always say, "I wish you could see yourself the way I see you." However, when I said "Will you still love me if I'm big and fat?" (I meant once I got pregnant—an unfair question for anybody to ask another person, I know!) I could never have expected his response: "I love you too much to let you get big and fat!" I definitely did not see that coming and must admit I started to spin a bit. But we all know how that relationship turned out, so let's move on.

As I've gotten older, I've grown tired of being preoccupied with achieving a certain standard of beauty. It's exhausting! And who decides what qualifies as beautiful, anyway? And how on earth does someone live up to it? And what happens when that face begins to change? I've heard people walk up to my girls and say, "Your mother—she used to be so beautiful." *Uh, hi! Not dead yet! I'm standing right here, and I think I actually look rather good thank you very much.* I've never wanted my daughters to see me fixate on my appearance, and I've tried to spare them from the self-flagellation that I've put myself through. I guess at some point I just decided that even if I didn't love what I saw in the mirror, I would at least stop telling others about it.

These days, if I find myself quietly lamenting something about my looks or I hear someone else doing the same, I'm often reminded of that 2013 viral Dove video, "Real Beauty Sketches: You're More Beautiful Than You Think," in which a group of women are paired off with people they'd just met. One at a time, each woman is called into a room, where a forensic sketch artist sits behind a curtain, and she's asked to describe her appearance. As the women describe their features, their focus is primarily on the negative, saying things like, "My chin protrudes when I smile" or "I have a fat, rounder face" or "I have a big forehead." Then the partner who has just met each woman is asked to describe her appearance to the same forensic artist. The partners inevitably offer very different observations. Instead of a protruding chin the partner would say "she had nice eyes that lit up when she spoke" or "she had a cute nose." Then the artist shows each woman the two portraits side by side. The pictures based on self-descriptions generally show the women looking sadder, harsher, and more closed off. The portraits based on strangers' input depict faces that appear happier and more approachable—and they are also more accurate. It's a tearjerker, that video, but I think about it all the time. It's such an insightful way to showcase how distorted our self-image can be. By the end of the video, each of the women is in (or close to) tears, because they've realized how poorly they see themselves. Or maybe they're struck by seeing their beauty through someone else's eyes, or simply being the recipient of a stranger's kindness.

Over the years I've certainly learned that societal validation of your outside doesn't do much to change how you feel on the inside. But when someone you connect with and respect shares their view of you, and you can really hear it? That can have an impact.

Helena Christensen (yes, the *actual* supermodel) and I are close friends. Every time I see her, she talks about my butt. For years, I have gone to great lengths to disguise my curvy backside, or to make jokes about it, but she'll stand behind me and say "oooh look at that ass!" as if I have something she admires. And yes, of course it makes me feel good! She says it and she means it—she's not just flattering me—and when I wear a bit of a tighter dress and wonder if I'm making the wrong choice, I try to allow her voice in my head to drown out all the critical ones.

Does that mean I revel in seeing my naked self in the mirror? Not so much. It's a bit of a surprise every time—I expect to see twentysomething Brooke's tight abs, but fiftysomething Brooke's much looser tummy is staring back at me. When I picture myself in my head, I still see that younger version of me. And studies show that adults forty and over, on average, feel about 20 percent younger than we actually are.[2] Has anyone ever asked you your age and you respond "thirty-five," before remembering that, oh, you're actually forty-five? Your mind hasn't quite caught up with the rest of you. It's called "subjective age," and the younger your subjective age, the better off you are. It can have a significant effect on physical and mental health, and go so far as to be predictive of life expectancy. But it can also make looking in the mirror a somewhat startling experience. What we see is just so misaligned with what we expect to see.

It was a result of my newfound strength and body confidence that the first inkling of this book, and of my business, Commence, hit me. I was walking down the beach one day with one of my best male friends, basking in the glory of actually feeling good about myself. "The irony of it all," I said, "is that I've been insecure my whole life. Now, I finally feel fit and strong in my own body—I'm proud of how I look, and more capable physically—and my life is less fraught and more consistently joyful. I feel lighter and ready to live my life. But the messaging I'm getting back is that by fifty, we're finished. I believe I still have so much more to give, yet I'm being turned down and overlooked and dismissed everywhere I go. It's like, 'you've had a good run, but now you've got one foot in the grave.'"

Sometimes it's easier to notice the physical changes in yourself than the emotional or mental ones, so even though much of my headspace had evolved over the last decade, this contrast between how I looked and felt physically and how society treated me was easier to spot. It felt glaring! And the biggest surprise of the whole thing was that I truly didn't see it coming. I was totally taken by surprise. Here I was assuming that because I felt good about myself for maybe the first time, the world would come and reward me for that. Isn't that what *The Secret* taught us? It seemed only fair. But as Chris often asks me, "Why do you think the world is fair?" I've been on this planet a long time, how could I have been so naive about the way it works?

Because all my closest friends were also in their fifties, I knew this wasn't a "Brooke Shields problem." It was a female one. The ladies in my life were all in a better place than they were in their twenties or thirties, but they also felt undervalued. It occurred to me that it's easy for an actress to bemoan not getting parts or beauty campaigns like she used to, but what about all the other women our age across the world? Those who are at home raising kids, or are (or are soon-to-be) empty nesters, or going to the office nine to five? Who is acknowledging *their* value? How is the world reacting to them these days? Where is the incentive to continue to move forward with pride?

"So why don't you do it?" my friend said.

"Do what?"

"Create a place to start the dialogue, to better understand

what others your age are feeling. Take the temperature of this demographic, build the community, and start the discussion."

The more I thought about it, the more I liked the idea: create a safe platform for women over forty to speak freely about how they feel and how this era is treating them.

It's a lofty goal, to try to get to the core of an entire generation, but I figured I could at least try to facilitate a dialogue. It's not like I launched a company the very next day, but that day on the beach is when the wheels started turning and I began thinking about the misunderstandings surrounding this era of life—about what it is, and what it can be.

Not too long after that day, I broke my femur, and of course my workouts changed drastically. First came rehab—lots and lots of rehab. Then, when my physical abilities returned, my exercise became more focused on function. There was a time when the impetus behind all my exercise was *what will make me smaller?* Vanity was the primary driver. But getting skinnier is (finally!) no longer the goal. Strength and endurance and mobility and muscle quality—those are the pieces that will serve me as I age. If breaking the largest bone in my body taught me anything, it definitely taught me that. After all, I don't just want to be around to see my grandkids one day, I want to be able to get on the floor and play with them and then get back up on my own. I want to be able to pick them up without moaning and carry them across the park.

So instead of asking, What will make me smaller? I ask, What will keep me moving? And also, What will I enjoy?? And is there a marriage of the two? I enjoy dancing and going on long walks. I love Pilates. Can those be the exercises that accompany me into the next decade? The other day I walked from Forty-Fourth Street and Fifth Avenue down to the West Village, and by the time I got home I was drenched in sweat, but I was also thrilled to realize that, *Oh look, I got my workout in!* I don't particularly like going to the gym, but I know I need to factor in weight training, because again: health. Chris wants me to join him at his boxing workout, and I'm sure that if I did it every day for a few months I really would look amazing . . . but at what cost? Don't get me wrong, I like punching—it's a huge release—but I'm not that excited about the idea of learning boxing techniques. If this were twenty years ago I would have jumped at the chance to be seen as a tough girl in a gym packed with strong guys and actual boxers. But not today. I'll stick to activities I look forward to.

The joy of this phase of life isn't that you wake up one day fitter than ever—you don't. The years may earn you confidence and an ability to care less about what others think, but they won't magically reward you with strength or physical health. The fact that women lose 3 to 8 percent of muscle mass per decade after the age of thirty is just science. It is harder (not impossible!) to lose weight after forty, especially without the help of weight-loss drugs. Exercise plays a part in protecting our maturing bodies and our physical and mental health. So this is not a "do what you want! Who cares!" manifesto. Honestly, in the moments I've tried that, it didn't feel good. I've gone through periods where I've chosen sleep over exercise, I've decided to eat whatever I want and drink whatever I want because, screw it, it was the holidays or I just finished a big project and I wanted a break. But each time, I found myself a little bit worse off. I was more tired. I felt more uncomfortable in my body. I had less energy, was more down. But this doesn't need to be a time of pressure, either. For the first time, I feel inspired to work out how I want, in a way that makes me happy, because the end goals have changed. I could starve myself or work out constantly and take whatever diet drug is making the headlines this week, but what on earth for? Skinniness is not the holy grail to which I want to dedicate my time. Or my dollars. Neither is a procedure that takes all the years off my face. We all know how old I am, and no amount of Botox is ever going to change that. (Not that I'm against it. I'll admit that before a movie I'll get my frown line in my forehead touched up. We all make our choices.)

Lest I come off as preachy or—even worse—a hypocrite, let me be clear that I am not insisting that we all sit back and passively embrace all evidence of aging when there's something we truly don't like. But I've begun to shift my focus to what *I* feel comfortable with rather than what I assume will please others. For example, I still dye my roots. Perhaps one day I'll be ready to cut off my locks and embrace the gray—probably when I get tired of the time and expense necessary to keep my hair dark— but I'm not there yet. I love my brown, slightly highlighted hair. I also get Fraxels, which are basically laser treatments that help even out skin tone, because I like the effect it has on my face. Is the desire to have a face with fewer age spots a product of a society that puts too much emphasis on youth? Yes, I'm sure it is. But for now, it's a procedure that makes me feel better about my skin, without altering how I actually look. (At this point, my face is what it is—chasing an aesthetic to the point of becoming unrecognizable is not my goal.)

Also, I won't pretend for a second that I've thrown caution to the wind when it comes to getting photographed. When paparazzi snap me—which they do all the time, even as I'm walking my dog—I still prefer to look put together.

One day last year Taylor Swift was at Bradley Cooper's house in my neighborhood (my Swiftie daughters begged me to pop over and say hi, but as I pointed out, I wasn't invited, nor did I suspect Taylor had a burning desire to meet this then fifty-eight-year-old actress). Hordes of photographers gathered near my house, hoping to capture the world's biggest superstar. But as they waited for her to emerge, they settled for me as I walked to the corner store. I knew that might happen, so I wore an outfit that I'd feel good sporting in the pages of *People*. After Taylor left, many of the photographers hung around, and when I returned from the store I joked with them that they decided to wait for the leftovers. A few of them blurted out, "We still love you, Brooke!" and I smiled. The "still" stung a bit, but I'm not upset that time passes. And the photos they got weren't half bad!

I'm all for each of us doing whatever we need to in order to truly feel better *about* ourselves, *for* ourselves. A close friend of mine recently had a face-lift after being bothered by certain areas of her eyes and jawline for years. I was happy for her because I knew how long she had felt dissatisfied. I hoped she was going to feel great afterward. When I said as much, she suggested that I couldn't relate. "Well, honey," she said, "you weren't born with a face that was going to need work." She wasn't trying to be unkind, but it struck me because it was another reminder that people assume I don't share their insecurities about jowls or heavy eyelids or deep lines that begin at my nostrils and crevice downward. Of course I do! I'm not ready to go under the knife anytime soon, but I'll keep finding alternatives to look my best. And we need to remove the shame associated with all of it. We shame women for not looking like they did as teens, and then shame them for any intervention they undergo to look younger. My friend asked me to keep her news in confidence, and I swore that I would, but I hoped it wasn't because she felt embarrassed. (And by the way, I'm not breaching that confidence, because I have more than a few friends who have had procedures, so this story could be about any one of them!) But we shouldn't have to hide these things. My mother had a face-lift when she was forty. The recovery was brutal, but eventually she healed and was glad she did it. She died at seventy-nine, and when I looked at her face toward the end of her life, I would have guessed she was in her late sixties. That would have made her happy.

I know there are people out there who take my aging face as a physical affront. If I don't look like the Brooke Shields that everyone knew and imprinted on, I've done something horribly wrong. I've come to accept that's more about them than me. My getting older is a reminder that they're getting older, and perhaps they haven't come to see their forties and fifties as the empowering rite of passage that I do. But despite what anyone else might prefer, mine is a fiftysomething face, and for now, I accept that. So instead of feeling tired and beaten down by the changes to my features, I try to think of myself as a more detailed painting. I may try to give myself a little restorative touch-up from time to time, but I don't want to erase the detail entirely. These lines are here because I've laughed and lived.

There's a novel I often think about, called *Angle of Repose*, by Wallace Stegner. The title comes from the term for the steepest angle at which soil or rocks can slope without beginning to slide or slump. It's the positioning of perfect balance—somewhere between rest and effort, the angle at which the snow sits piled on a mountain without sliding into an avalanche. The metaphor has always stuck with me, and it's the notion I keep at the forefront of my mind as I settle into this phase of my life. What is my personal angle of repose? Everyone's is different, I imagine. For me, it's not killing myself at the gym every day or obsessing over my looks at the expense of my mental health or self-worth, but it's not ignoring those things entirely either. It involves doing something physical that keeps my blood pumping and my muscles working and helps prevent osteoporosis. It's engaging in something where I have to push myself from time to time but is also fun, or at least fun-*ish*. I don't want to settle so deeply into the "letting myself go" that it harms me rather than helps; but I also don't want to feel so much pressure to maintain the body and face I had as a teen that I prioritize those things over enjoyment. I want to feel good about my appearance if I bump into someone I know on the street, while knowing that if I get caught in an unflattering photo, it doesn't change anything about my worth or who I am. I want to settle into the middle place, where there's effort in the comfort, and comfort in the effort. Where I can accept myself and love myself, but yes, still find my best angles and, without a doubt, the optimal lighting! I meant what I said—I'm a work in progress just like anyone else. And thank God for that. It's far more fun than thinking you have it all figured out.

7

Coming in Hot

A MENOPAUSE MANIFESTO

In April 2016, I was in Savannah, Georgia, filming *Daisy Winters*, a movie in which I played a mother battling cancer. One evening we were shooting a scene where I had to pick up my eleven-year-old daughter from a police station. I was wearing a long brown suede jacket, and while we waited to start filming, I sat in a car outside the station. It was springtime in the South, and I was wearing a heavy coat in a car, so I was already hot—but all of a sudden, I found myself absolutely dripping in sweat. It was as if (warm) water was being poured down my forehead, to the point that I thought maybe I was dying. I was playing a character who *was* dying, but I am not a method actor, so this was not how I had prepared for the role.

I truly didn't know what was going on, but whatever it was, I knew I didn't like it. I am a professional. I don't delay filming. I'm not late to set. I don't come unprepared. I never make my problems anyone else's business. So when my body failed to get the memo, and it affected everyone (the flop sweat was so thick that no movie magic or special effects could hide it on-screen), I was rattled. We had to stop shooting until I cooled off, because the makeup artist couldn't mop me down fast enough. It was acutely embarrassing. Plus, we were in a time crunch because it was a night shoot. The whole cast and crew had already worked a ten-hour day and were approaching that dangerous point that would veer us into overtime. Keep in mind, this was not a high-budget film but an indie that needed every penny the director had raised. Now I was not only worried about my sweat but also that I was costing the film money . . . which, of course, only made me more anxious and sweatier. I kept saying "I'm so sorry, I'm so sorry, I don't know what's happening, I'm so embarrassed. I hope I'm not sick!"

On film sets, a common trick to cool down after a long day under the hot lights is to dip a suede shammy in ice-cold water mixed with Sea Breeze astringent and rest it on your neck. I did that, and the whole crew (and the cast in my scene) waited me out. Eventually we picked up filming. Still, I couldn't stop apologizing. Afterward the director, who, like me, was a fifty-year-old woman, turned to me and said, "It might just be . . . something that happens to women?" *Hint, hint.*

Perhaps it should have already occurred to me that I was having my first hot flash, but truly, it did not. The calendar said I was fifty, sure, but I didn't *feel* fifty. I didn't live like a fifty-year-old. I didn't act like one! I'm not sure what I thought fifty-year-olds uniformly looked like or acted like—more lined, more tired, more decrepit, I guess. But even as I hit the milestone birthday I was in a bit of denial. I loved turning forty, but fifty sounded old. I hadn't yet realized that all my preconceived notions of what that age represented were rooted in myths rather than reality, and as a result my hope had been to ignore the birthday altogether. It was my assistant at the time who insisted, "You have great kids, a great life, you look amazing. You should celebrate yourself!" He convinced me to throw a party at the Refinery Rooftop, which had an incredible view of the Empire State Building, and the truth is I'm glad he did. We had swing dancers and tequila and tacos, Chris and my girls gave speeches (well, Grier, who was nine at the time, recited two original poems . . . or as she pronounced it, "poe-emmmmmms"), and there was something so heartwarming about seeing my friends from high school and college and adulthood all in one place.

Now, eleven months later, I was reminded why I'd wanted to ignore my transition into this new decade. When my *Daisy Winters* director implied that maybe I was beginning to go through "the change," my first thought, aside from *I'm definitely not old enough*, was, *Is this for real?? After everything I've gone through . . . this is the reward?* I wasn't ready to start going downhill. My vibrant, still-filming-movies life certainly didn't feel like it was at the beginning of the end. But because I'd only ever heard negative things about menopause, I assumed that gloom and doom awaited me. Certainly, that was the cultural narrative around menopause at the time: *Once you can't have babies, you're dried-up and your usefulness wanes.* (It was either that, or menopause would make you go "street-rat crazy," as a 2009 Jack in the Box ad so eloquently put it.)

Plus, this particular hot flash came at a moment when I felt like so much was coming together for me: I hadn't done a movie in a while and I was really proud of the performance I was giving in *Daisy Winters*. It was empowering to be back at work, and I was enjoying the independence of being on a movie set after taking time off from long projects in order to be with my kids. I had a real "back at it" pep in my step until I was knocked out at the knees by this blaring alarm bell that seemed to be signaling "Alert! Alert! It's all over for you now!!" I was also working with Sterling Jerins, then an eleven-year-old actress who was the exact age I was when I did *Pretty Baby*. Playing her mother felt full circle and symbolic but also a little bit God-giveth-and-God-taketh-away. I just remember thinking, *Oh right, that's how life works.*

I hadn't given much thought to menopause before this moment. It just wasn't on my radar, which is maybe strange but, I've also learned, entirely common. Studies have shown that most women are completely in the dark about this stage—or have only minimal knowledge about it—before the age of forty.[1] The most popular source of menopause information or education, according to that study, are friends and the internet—not doctors. In fact, one survey found that two-thirds of women ages forty to sixty-four said they've *never* discussed menopause with a health care provider.[2] *Never!* In another study of postmenopausal women, more than 60 percent said they only sought out information about menopause when they started experiencing symptoms themselves.[3] And of those going through menopause, only about 25 percent reported getting any treatment for their symptoms.[4]

It's not just patients who feel uninformed. Studies show that plenty of doctors feel ill-equipped to discuss menopause, which is probably why patients feel underserved. I've mentioned already that one-fifth of medical residents report having received not a single lecture on menopause. (If you need evidence that women of a certain age are generally ignored, look no further.) A Mayo Clinic survey of medical residents found that "just 7 percent of new physicians in family medicine and gynecology felt adequately prepared to deal with patients' menopause."[5] This, despite estimates that there will be about 1.1 billion menopausal women worldwide by the year 2025. I don't think you need a psychology degree to know that the more we avoid talking about something, the scarier it seems.

My ignorance about menopause in large part resulted from a lack of education or conversations with doctors, but I think I also presumed that given all I'd gone through with IVF and postpartum depression, nothing could be worse. All three—in vitro fertilization, postpartum depression, and menopause—involve hormonal fluctuations that can result in similar side effects. I took Lupron when I was doing IVF (the same drug my father was taking for cancer at the time), and the side effects involved constant sweating and mood swings, so by the time menopause entered my consciousness, I figured I'd already been through a dress rehearsal.

Luckily, the hot flash on the set of *Daisy Winters* was a bit of a one-off, at least for a while. I was not plagued daily or monthly by hot flashes after that, though I did begin to notice that extreme situations—pitching a project or performing in front of a large crowd or even just talking about something emotional—would trigger a sweating episode. My friend Lisa and I used to tell each other we were "having a wee bit of the peri," because by then we both knew we were in perimenopause, that lovely transitional state before actual menopause, which can stretch anywhere from a few years to a decade. (Menopause is defined as not having a period for twelve months. The years of waning estrogen and irregular periods and, yes, occasional hot flashes leading up to that twelve-month marker are perimenopause.)

A year or two after the *Daisy Winters* episode, when night sweats and wrestling with the bedsheets became a more regular part of my life, I brought it all up with my gynecologist for the first time. She started me on bioidenticals—estrogen and progesterone—in order to, as she described it, help me get over the hump so I wasn't plummeting off a cliff. The intention was that these hormones would help me avoid the most severe menopause symptoms: the even more extreme hot flashes and mood swings and insomnia and dryness and changes to hair and skin. Obviously, whether or not to take hormones is a personal decision, but for me, low doses of hormones have been incredibly helpful. I take them sublingually, rather than a pill, and they have kept me a little more even-keeled through this phase. Of course, this was my individual experience. There are plenty of other options—both pharmaceutical and homeopathic—and a woman should consult her physician about what makes sense for her. But I do think these hormones have eased my transition, because I've got to be honest, the actual experience of menopause, for me, has not been that bad.

I want to be clear that everyone's experience is different. Just as every woman's period is different—some people get debilitating cramps, others float through that time of the month with a couple of super-plus tampons and they're on their way—so, too, is their transition away from having a period. But menopause is a phase, and it's one that we can navigate. Do you remember getting your period for the first time? A nightmare! You had to figure out how to put in a tampon or apply a bulky pad. To decide if you could go swimming or wear white jeans. Then there are the other hormonal changes. Pregnancy is pretty wild. Breast-feeding? More than wild. Over the course of our lives, we get used to changes like these, which all can be incredibly difficult. There's always something you need to figure out, but that's our baseline. As women, there is no biological phase that doesn't come without challenges. Menopause is another change—"the puberty of midlife," as Dr. Suzanne Gilberg-Lenz, author of *Menopause Bootcamp*, calls it—and we get through it. Like any phase, it has negatives and positives.

For me, one of the hardest parts of the transition was accepting the finality of my fertility. It's not like I was planning to have another baby at fifty, but potential is a powerful drug. I spent so much of my life looking forward to having a big family. And yes, I had an incredibly difficult year after Rowan was born, but for the most part, when I was a new mom I reveled in it, soaking up my babies' sweet little faces and cuddling with them. Becoming a mother was such a profound accomplishment for me. When I struggled to get pregnant, I beat myself up so relentlessly, and I did so because I felt flawed in some fundamental way. Carrying those two little girls inside my body made me feel normal. It made me feel important! I loved having a bigger body, and a bigger *purpose* to my body. For so much of my life, I felt like my body—even my fertility—belonged to other people. Having my beautiful babies gave me a sense of ownership again.

After Grier was born, I thought very seriously about having a third child. If I'd started when I was younger, I probably would have gone through with it. (I'm glad I never got pregnant with my first husband because it would have been a disaster. When we got divorced he made that very clear. "Be thankful we didn't have children," he said, "because I would not have made this easy for you." *Well, thank you for that tidbit*, I thought. *You just made this particular transition much easier!*) I went to the doctor when Grier was a toddler to discuss IVF, but by then I was in my midforties. My OB-GYN said it was possible but cautioned me about all the very real risks at my age, and I started to think, *Maybe I should leave well enough alone. I have two healthy daughters, I don't need to push it.* It was hard to fully come to terms with the idea that I had no more pregnancies to look forward to, though, and it hurt to let that door close. I mourned that loss for quite some time.

But while aging into menopause brought grief about the babies I would never have, I also gained a sense of appreciation for my daughters, now that they were young adults. We were entering new life stages together, and I didn't want to get so caught up in the loss of fertility that I overlooked what I was gaining: two amazing young women who I could connect with on a more adult level. In fact, my girls were getting their periods just as I was losing mine, which felt symbolic in itself. They were bursting into their womanhood as a piece of mine was coming to its conclusion.

And there are indeed some good aspects of menopause. Not having a period is, in a word, freedom. In the second season of *Fleabag*, Kristin Scott Thomas, whose character has just won a "woman in business" award, gives an incredible monologue, explaining to Phoebe Waller-Bridge's title character why fifty-eight is so much better than thirty-three: "[Women] have pain on a cycle for years and years and then, just when you feel you are making peace with it all, what happens? The menopause comes—the fucking menopause comes!—and it is the most wonderful fucking thing in the world. And yes, your entire pelvic floor crumbles and you get fucking hot and no one cares. But then you're free! No longer a slave, no longer a machine with parts. You're just a person, in business."

For my podcast, I interviewed *Menopause Bootcamp* author Gilberg-Lenz, and she shared about her own experience going through menopause. It was, to say the least, not the story we usually hear: "I know myself so much better [now]," she said. "We feel so identified with our cycle because we spend so many decades in it, avoiding it, managing it, whatever. And then it's like, who are we without a cycle? And guess what? I really like who I am without a cycle! It turns out I was affected by my hormones in ways that I didn't even really realize. And I feel just more steady. I feel more like myself. I feel more calm. I'm a pretty intense person, so I'm not as emotional in a way that bothers *me*. And I'm super creative. I'm digging into that creativity in a whole new way. It has been amazing."

Not dealing with cramps and bleeding and birth control and worrying if you've somehow leaked through your tampon and stained your pants—there's relief in that. Biology is so hard on women that I'm honestly surprised we don't just get a period forever, but eventually with no eggs. Bleeding forever, without the fertility . . . that's how I'd figure nature would do it. Of course, there's so much biology I can't wrap my head around. Why is it that men can procreate into their seventies, whereas women have a shelf life? There's something fundamentally unjust about that. And yet for so long, we are the ones who are slaves to our bodies. First your period, and then when you get pregnant it's as if you're invaded by aliens. Once you have a baby, your milk-filled breasts will start to leak through any breast pads if so much as a stranger's baby begins to cry! That is incredible to me. The whole thing is totally bizarre if you think too much about it—and then you're done and . . . that's it. You're an "empty vessel," and suddenly ignored. Finding myself in that life stage is when I really started to think, *Wait a minute, I did not make it through all that bullshit just to be told that I'm no longer of value.* Once I went through menopause myself, it was so much more glaring how ridiculous this notion is that you're on your way to death just because you're no longer fertile. I was not going to be reduced to that.

I'm not trying to sugarcoat what is a very real and significant physiological change. I know that it can be quite difficult, both physically and emotionally. But I also know that it's not a big bad wolf waiting to devour you. It's not this looming thing we all need to be deathly afraid of. Research shows that perimenopausal and postmenopausal women (who can still experience symptoms up to ten years after the transition) have more positive attitudes toward menopause than premenopausal women (who, in one study, most commonly described their attitude toward menopause as one of "dread"[6]). In other words, those who are currently in the throes of perimenopause or have already been through it don't feel so horribly about it. And between those who are postmenopausal and perimenopausal, the postmenopausal have more positive attitudes. In a study literally titled "It's Not as Bad as You Think,"[7] researchers found, well, just that. Women went through menopause, and while it certainly could be difficult, they felt more neutral or accepting toward it than those who hadn't made the transition. Humans have a tendency to "overestimate the intensity and duration of emotional reactions to future events," according to that study, and menopause is no exception. Those who don't know what to expect—or who've collected their information from media portrayals—assume it will be horrible. But the lack of information on menopause doesn't negatively affect just *attitudes* toward menopause, it also affects the actual *experience*. Studies show that more education and knowledge about menopause is correlated with a better quality of life when you're going through it.

What else can improve the experience of menopause? Sharing about it! "For people who go through [menopause] in a community of other women who are sharing advice and support and have tools that are useful and beneficial and validated, it's a completely different experience, just like any other experience we go through with loved ones and with our girlfriends," Dr. Gilberg-Lenz told me. "Honestly, we get through it. We get through the breakups, we get through the job losses, we get through the changes in our lives. We get through the pregnancies, the lack of pregnancies . . . and when we get to the other side, here's the awesome thing: there's this incredible liberation. There's this unleashing of creativity, of recognition of our own power and agency."

The science bears out Dr. Gilberg-Lenz's point. Social support has been shown to improve the menopausal experience for women and reduce the risk of mental health disorders in women going through this transition. No big surprise—going through any major life shift without being able to talk to other people about it is hard. My battle with postpartum depression was most challenging when I was suffering in silence—once I was able to open up about it and get some support, I was on my way to recovery.

The good news is that conversations around menopause are

undoubtedly picking up, with many notable women leading the charge. Oprah did a whole class on it as part of her online "The Life You Want" series, in conversation with Drew Barrymore, Gayle King, and Maria Shriver. Naomi Watts, the founder of Stripes, a "menopause solutions brand," has developed products that address symptoms like dryness and thinning hair. In early 2024, Halle Berry's wellness company, Re-Spin, announced they were going to focus more specifically on menopause. Jill Biden has spoken up about the importance of advancing menopause research, and so has Michelle Obama. Not to mention that it's also becoming big business: venture capital firms invested more than $500 million in menopause care from 2015 to 2023,[8] and the menopause market is projected to reach more than $24 billion by 2030.[9]

That menopause is finally becoming a hot topic (I know, sorry) is undoubtedly a powerful development. It's unfortunate that it took the promise of a financial upside to bring it into mainstream conversation, but however we come by it, dialogue should destigmatize the experience and empower women with information and resources. Perhaps most important, it may inspire more research, which scientists say is critically necessary. Questions remain about whether environmental factors can influence menopause, how different stages of menopause affect chronic health conditions or cardiovascular health or brain health, and why some women experience severe symptoms while others have barely any at all. We also need more studies on hormone therapy and other potential interventions. According to an editorial in the scientific journal *Nature*, "At least in the United States, it is difficult to track funding for menopause research, because the NIH hasn't assigned menopause a unique identification code like the ones other conditions (such as anorexia or prostate cancer) have. Someone wanting to find out must read every grant that mentions 'menopause' and add up the numbers manually."[10] Happily, some progress is being made. In May 2024, a group of bipartisan women senators, joined by Halle Berry, introduced the Advancing Menopause Care and Mid-Life Women's Health Act, which would authorize $275 million over five years to boost research, training, awareness, and education around "menopause and mid-life women's health issues." Finally, something both parties can get behind!

But while more menopause talk is a step in the right direction, I still believe the *way* we talk about it could use some improvement. We tend to focus only on the negative. And while yes, there are some distinctly negative symptoms, when they become the focus of the conversation, it's no wonder that it's hard to find a silver lining. There is no reverence, no admiration, no respect surrounding this life stage. Only fear or mocking. That probably shouldn't come as much of a surprise—women's reproductive value has been the source of mockery and attacks for at least a century, probably longer. Expressions like "she's on the rag" (because before disposable pads, women actually used rags) or "it's that time of the month" don't exactly paint a kind or generous picture. But it's hard to change attitudes toward this phase—to remind the world of our value and relevance and energy—when our dialogue around it is still full of horror or disdain. At Commence, we're working on a hair-care line, and one of those products is an "instant" shampoo, because I won't call it a "dry" shampoo. We get to a certain age and everything is all about dryness, and, sorry, but that's not all I am! And menopause, too, is not all I am. It's a part of this life stage, and it's one that hasn't been taken nearly seriously enough, but it's not the entirety.

When I said that I was launching a space for women from ages forty to sixty to find a community, people often thought I was speaking in code. That "find a community" was a euphemism for "talk about menopause." But we are more than our menstrual cycles, or lack thereof. This phase of life is about many things—our bodies are one piece, but so are relationships and careers and emotional growth and creativity. You'd think that all goes without saying, and yet here we are, always focused on this one big change. Menopause is a physiological stage of life. It comes with obstacles. But it is not who you are.

I don't get my period anymore. I'm still taking hormones. I'm still talking with my doctor to make sure my current prescriptions make sense for me, and tinkering with them from time to time so that my hormones and temperament and sex drive are where we want them to be. (If you are dealing with any symptoms of menopause and they are causing you discomfort, discuss them with your doctor! There is no reason to suffer in silence, and this notion that women should just "deal with it" is outdated and, well, absurd.) I have gone through plenty of changes—physically, emotionally, and mentally—in the past decade. But also, in the past six decades! Human beings are constantly changing. Some of my most recent changes are due to menopause, sure. But some are just due to getting older and maybe (definitely!) wiser. Some are just me, as a human being, evolving, becoming stronger and more confident in myself and my opinions. I'll admit I got a bit more irritable and lost a bit of patience at times. "You're so edgy, Mom," my kids would say, not in the complimentary way. Maybe my exasperation *was* hormonal. Or maybe I'm just more resolved in my stance on things. Maybe I don't have the same patience for bullshit. Maybe time doesn't feel as endless as it once did, so using it wisely feels more urgent. It's hard to pick a culprit. It's probably a little bit of all of the above. We are complex creatures, and that only gets truer as the years go by.

8

I'll Be There for You

THE ONE WITH A NEW BEST FRIEND

used to love watching *Nightcap*. The sitcom, which aired on Pop TV for two seasons in 2016 and 2017, starred Ali Wentworth as Staci Cole, the head talent booker at the fictional nighttime talk show *Nightcap with Jimmy*. Ali was not just the star but the creator and one of the writers, and the scripts were clever and skewering and dark (my favorite kind of comedy). Each episode featured celebrity guests playing themselves. Jimmy, the host of the show, is never actually seen on-screen—the episodes revolve around his staff's interactions with that evening's celebrity guests. Sarah Jessica Parker, Gwyneth Paltrow, Michael J. Fox, and Paul Rudd all appeared in the first season.

I didn't know Ali well at the time—I'd met her socially in a casual way—but after watching a couple of episodes, I knew I wanted to appear on the show. Not long before the first season finale, I sent her a cold email. "You don't really know me," I said, "but I think you are one of the funniest people and one of the best writers out there, and I'd love to work with you. I know I can do it—I've seen the actors coming through your show and I'd really like to be one of them."

She probably responded with more than three words but

what I remember of her note back to me was, "Are you serious?" I guess she was surprised to be hearing from me.

"Absolutely," I said. "I've come to a point in my life where I've learned it doesn't hurt to ask for what I want and put it out into the universe." My only caveat, I explained, was that I really hoped she would ask the most of me. Writers tend to play it safe when they're creating a part for me. I don't know if they're worried about offending me or they don't think I can handle a tough role or they assume I won't have a sense of humor, but I like surprising people (both writers *and* audiences), so I asked Ali to please challenge me. About three months later, she wrote me a note and said she'd finished the episode.

"I'll do it!" I said.

"But you haven't even read it yet," she responded.

"I trust you," I wrote. "I'm in."

In my episode, I play a borderline-psychotic version of myself. I force Ali's character, Staci, to drink with me before the show, and then rope the episode's other guest star, *Gossip Girl's* Kelly Rutherford, into joining us as well. It gets increasingly more sinister—I do that knife trick where I quickly stab the table between my fingers and then threaten to punch "Goody Two-shoes" Kelly in the face. Then, when she passes out drunk and we think she's dead, I make Staci help me roll her up in a rug to dispose of the body. This is all while continually reminding Staci that I am "Hollywood icon Brooke Shields. I AM America's sweetheart!"

I loved the script Ali wrote so much—my role really was so over-the-top and had so much "crazy Brooke" in it—that I made sure to come ready. I had a lot of dialogue, but we got through it quickly. All my scenes were opposite Ali, and we fell into an almost effortless rhythm. Something about our comedic timing and chemistry just *worked*, and while that doesn't always translate off-screen or mean you are going to be friends, it was clear from the beginning that we had a mutual respect and admiration for each other.

At the end of the day of shooting, Ali admitted I surprised her. "I didn't know what to expect, but, man, you came armed and ready and flexible and fucking funny," she said. "Nobody knows how funny you are!"

Unbeknownst to Ali, she had said the magic words. I love comedy. Making people laugh *matters* to me. I'm not a stand-up comic, I don't tell jokes, but I say what's on my mind, and when people laugh it's like they get me. Howard Stern, Wanda Sykes, Garry Shandling, Larry David, Whoopi Goldberg, David Spade, Matthew Perry . . . to make people like that laugh, it gives me joy. It's such a rush.

I've always enjoyed making people laugh but I don't know that anyone acknowledged my comedic talent until I appeared on *Friends* in 1996. I remember getting the call to be a guest star on "The One After the Super Bowl." I said yes immediately, also before reading the script. All I could think was, *God, I hope I make them laugh.* Like the rest of the world, I was obsessed with *Friends* and was excited and honored to have been asked to be a part of it. I was worried they'd want me to play myself and was relieved when, instead, I was asked to play Joey's crazy stalker date, Erika.

I flew to Los Angeles to tape the episode. I had never done a sitcom and was nervous and very quiet the first day. The second day of rehearsals I had a scene with the whole group, and I watched as the cast shared all these inside jokes that made them laugh hysterically. I ached to be included but was just a day player and not part of the inner circle. They weren't being rude at all, they were just a close-knit cast with funny memories and private jokes. I was a onetime character. Still, I yearned for them to like me and think I was funny. But how? It was as if making The Friends laugh was more important than what I was going to do with the part. I watched their banter and tried not to intrude, but all of a sudden my "in" occurred to me.

Matthew Perry had this one bit where he would take a running start and, as if sliding into home base, he'd throw himself on the floor in front of a pretty girl and pretend to look up her skirt. It seemed as if he had done this particular bit hundreds of times, and it never failed to get the others to laugh. Well, during a short break from rehearsing the final scene in Joey's living room, I decided to take my chance. I casually walked away to the opposite side of the sound stage and then turned back suddenly, broke into a full run, and headed straight to where Matt was standing. I dove to the carpet at his feet, pulled up the bottom of one of his pant legs, and pretended to peek up his pants. The friends were stunned into silence—nobody really knew what was happening. Lying on the floor, I had a moment of sheer panic. *Nice move, Brooke*, I thought. *Who do you think you are to try to make the cast of one of the funniest shows of all time laugh! You suck, and now you're going to get fired!* (I'd heard that guests got fired all the time, as early as after the first read-through of the script.) After what felt like thirty minutes, but which was, in actuality, only about three seconds, Matthew burst into hysterics, saying, "I can't believe you just did that! That was the funniest thing ever!" Once he broke the ice, the rest of the cast began to laugh, and I was able to breathe. Of course, that's when I began to feel the pain of the rug burns on my knees and elbows. But it was all worth it. To make Matthew laugh, it was the sweetest thing.

That afternoon the cast invited me to have lunch with them at the fancy commissary and go to the gym on the lot. I had made it in Hollywood! And in the episode itself, my willingness to embrace the crazy and go hard for the laugh made an impression, too. The day after the show aired, I got the call asking me to star in my very own sitcom, *Suddenly Susan*.

But twenty years after that episode filmed, Ali was right. *Suddenly Susan* stopped airing in 2000, and in the time since I hadn't had many opportunities to remind fans—or the industry—of my comedic chops. I think she admired how committed I was to the role she wrote for me, and how willing and unfettered I was. I admired how smart and talented she was. Not to mention that we were around the same age, with kids about the same age. After filming our *Nightcap* episode, Ali and I started hanging out, and we just clicked. We also realized we shared a similar sensibility about life in the entertainment industry. We'd often find ourselves at a fancy party, she nursing a cranberry and soda and me with some form of tequila, both naturally falling into an Abbott-and-Costello, Lucy-and-Ethel shtick. Believe it or not, neither of us is totally comfortable with the chatter or opulence that can come with certain grand affairs. We find ourselves settling into these roles pretty regularly—we have this yin-and-yang banter we love. She's the self-deprecating one, I'm a bit looser and dorkier. Ali, George, and I did a panel for the *Pretty Baby* documentary when it came out and someone asked me a question, I can't remember what, and I began to answer and Ali interjected and we just went back and forth for a while until the moderator said, "George, the next question is for you," and he said, "Really? You don't want to keep watching this?" It's not that we're constantly *on* in a "Waka Waka" song-and-dance sense, but it's just easy. To be honest, not since meeting David Strickland, my late best male friend who I met on the set of *Suddenly Susan*, have I had a dynamic like this with someone.

Ali and I met when I was fifty. We laugh together, yes, but we've also been through the tough stuff, which is surely a function of our age. There were my seizure and femur break. Our kids leaving for college, which was a celebratory rite of passage but also pretty tough at times. She lost her brother and her father recently. People often ask how long we've known each other, and I'll just say, "Not long enough to merit how close we are." But the hard times can bind you.

I won't deny that I was surprised to develop such a close friendship in this phase of my life. I guess I didn't think it was possible. I already had a bestie from high school. Can you meet another, different kind of best girlfriend, later in life? I guess so. It feels like a version of falling in love again—and that's something you might not expect to happen in your fifties. Although apparently this phenomenon isn't unique to me. According to one study,[1] older adults have more close friendships than younger people do. Doesn't that seem counterintuitive? When you're young, you're surrounded by so many friends and acquaintances. I guess with time, though, we really connect with our people. The same study also found that adults fifty and older were more likely to be highly satisfied with their friendships than were their younger counterparts. I think, as we get older, quality matters more, and we just don't have time for relationships that aren't additive to our lives.

One of the best things about making friends in this era, I've found, is that those friends have *only* known you in this era. As much fun as shared history can be, sometimes it can also keep you stuck in the past. Friends from high school or college will always remember the person you were back then, and sometimes (oftentimes?) they assume you haven't changed. Or maybe they haven't changed in ways you wish they had. New friends come with no preconceived notions, and no baggage. Of course, Ali had some knowledge of who I was when we first met—and I knew some basic facts about her—but she didn't presume to know my insecurities or neuroses or hold behaviors against me that I'd long since outgrown.

Here's the truth: I am a little bit torn when it comes to friendship these days. Part of me wants to limit my circle. Maintaining friendships requires time and effort, and to be completely honest it can sometimes feel like my dance card is already very full. By the time my kids reached high school, I felt like I could confidently say I didn't need any new friends. I had childhood friends and college friends and people I'd met through work and raising kids. I was good. The other part of me knows I should invest in friendships—old and new—and wants to. After all, Ali has become one of the most important people in my life, and our friendship is enough proof to me that it's worth it to stay open to new connections even at this age.

There's also a bunch of research that shows friendships are tied not only to happiness but also to health and longevity as we age. In one study, people over fifty took a survey three times over eight years. Those who had high-quality friendships were 24 percent less likely to die during that span![2] Robert Waldinger, director of the Harvard Study of Adult Development and coauthor of *The Good Life*, has said the most unexpected finding of his study was how far-reaching the impact of friendship was for older people: "The people who were happiest, who stayed healthiest, and who lived the longest, were the people who had the warmest connections. In fact, good relationships were the strongest predictor of who was going to be happy and healthy as they grew old." It appears to me that this might be one area where women have a leg up. Friendships between men just seem to be different from those between women. At least, that seems to be the case in the heterosexual men's friendships that I've seen. As my husband puts it, "we don't sit around talking about feelings." But good friendships can literally be lifesavers.

Where I've landed is that I'm much more intentional about friendships at this age. I try not to spend as much time with the friends who generally exhaust me (we all have them, even if they mean well), and dedicate more energy to the relationships that feel mutually beneficial. In my younger years, I was less discerning. I felt obligated to give everyone equal time and ran myself ragged. At this age, you really start needing the good people, and quite frankly, I've become more stoic with anybody who doesn't gel with my life (sometimes I worry I take it to an extreme . . . there are people that I feel fairly repelled by now). On the other hand, I think I've also gotten needier with the real friends. The little girl in me still comes out sometimes and thinks, *Am I your best friend?? Do you really like me?* Because the people I value and care about and want to grow old with are becoming that much more precious to me.

Giving myself permission to prioritize friendships based on how they make me feel, as opposed to who I *should* be loyal to or who I feel obligated to talk to or what other people will think of my behavior? That didn't come easily.

Of course, I'm still learning, and sometimes I still act out of obligation. These days, when it comes to social events, my response tends to fall into one of three categories: one, "It's a no-brainer, count me in." Then there's the "I really don't want to go, but I should" category. In that case, sometimes I say yes and sometimes I don't, but I tend to have FOMO if I don't attend. When that happens, I try to balance the anticipation of feeling left out with an honest investigation of how I want to spend my time. *You don't get to have it both ways, Brooke*, I tell myself. I can either say yes and fully commit or say no and leave it at that. I can't say yes and then complain about it later or say no and then scroll Instagram feeling like nobody wants to play with me. And

I really try to adhere to that, which is worth something, because had social media been around when I was a teenager I would have definitely been on the scrolling-and-pouting train.

Then there is the third category, the one in which I know I definitely don't want to go to something, and I am relieved not to be invited. That at least feels like a little bit of growth. When I was younger I *always* wanted to be invited. I didn't genuinely want to be out and about all the time, but I was afraid of not being included. Now there are plenty of events or social gatherings where I might expect an invite but when I don't get it, I'm not personally affronted. Instead I'm a little bit grateful.

Even if FOMO and obligatory friendships still exist to some degree (age brings wisdom, sure, but old habits die hard), I'm happy to say there is one area where the drama of younger friendships really does level out as we age: competition and envy. When Ali and I get together with our daughters, one of my girls will always turn to me and say, "Mom, I hope I have a friendship like that when I'm older." Apparently, Ali's daughters have said the same. Seeing two strong women who lift each other up and have each other's backs and have an ease to their friendship, but who also still give each other shit and make each other laugh . . . it makes an impact on them. We all know what friendship can be like in adolescence. We know that *Mean Girls* might as well be a documentary. I love that our daughters get to see a model for female friendship that's about celebrating each other's accomplishments and reminding each other to bask in every little win. (Not to mention that Ali makes fun of me for all the same reasons my daughters make fun of me, which in turn makes them admire our relationship that much more.) There is a real beauty in midlife friendships, specifically in terms of lifting each other up. Not that any of my friends were explicitly at each other's throats or plagued with jealousy in the past, but there was often an element of keeping an eye on what others were doing and trying to keep up. Maybe it's biological. At this age, we're not all competing for the one male lion.

I also think I've gotten better at realizing that not every bump in the road is my fault. When someone is behaving in a way I don't like, or if they treat me in a way I don't like, I can usually see pretty clearly that it's about them, not me. I used to hold everyone to such a high standard, which would result in me getting hurt or disappointed sometimes. I couldn't understand why everyone didn't live up to this version of what I believed loyalty and friendship should look like. It was very black-and-white. Now I'm more confident meeting people where they are, with no desire to change them or "improve" their performance as a friend. It protects me from being disappointed, and from holding people to unfair standards. I know what I need of friends, but I put most of the expectations on myself—how I want to show up for people, and for whom. I like to believe I'm a very devoted friend, but I'm devoted to fewer people, and I don't feel the need to commit to everyone.

When I met Ali, she had a whole group of close friends. If the revolving door of A-listers on *Nightcap* was any indication, she clearly had not just a deep Rolodex of stars but strong relationships with them as well. Since we've become close she's made an effort to bring me into that fold. Of course I appreciate that, and I've met and become friends with some wonderful and fascinating people. But at this stage of my life, I no longer feel left out when my friends have other unique friendships or groups of friends with whom I am not as close. I met this group of women recently and they had a nickname for their group, "the clique" or "the club" or something, and all I could think was, *I do not want a jacket that says Pink Ladies.* I no longer crave that sense of belonging to a group in the way I once did.

In fact, instead of having one solid group of friends, I've found that I prefer to have little pockets here and there. I have a number of different friendships that fuel and nurture me in different ways. I have the athletic friend and the deep-talks friend and the party friend and the antiquing friend. I have friends who span ages, I have female friends and male friends, and I have, as Chris calls them, my "gay husband" friends. I connect with each one differently, and it's become clear to me as I age that I need this diversity of people in my life.

The ways in which friendships—and how we approach them—evolve with age is especially apparent to me now because my daughters are at the time in their lives where these relationships are so critical to them, but in an entirely different way. For example, they want to go to clubs when all I want to do is sit at someone's house for dinner. But on a more emotional level, I hear my daughters talking about mean girls or people who've talked shit behind their backs, and they take it to heart in such an intense way. You can't make someone grow up any faster, but when I hear about these interactions I just want to shake them and say, "You will so quickly learn it's about them, not you." Instead, they try to jump through hoops to be friends with certain people, and it breaks my heart a little.

Grier recently left for college, and that transition comes with its own friendship changes. Before she left, she and her friends wanted to be together all the time. And they wanted not only their friends to stick together but also their families to be friends and the parents to be besties. It was a nice idea, but not usually that easy to make a reality. This has been another feather in the cap of my friendship with Ali. Not only do we hit it off individually but—the rarest of things—we also mesh as couples and families. Chris and George like to discuss the headlines—I have never met anyone as smart as George, there is nobody in the world he hasn't interviewed or couldn't go head-to-head with—but Chris also makes George laugh, which is such a delight to watch. And Ali and Chris have their own comedic alliance. I know, it sounds like *The Hunger Games*, but there's no other way to describe it. It was kind of scary to me at first—we were together, all eight of us, and I was a bit intimidated by how quickly their minds work. I have never had a girlfriend who has been able to spar with Chris like that. It's on another level. But it's also such a joy, because we can be together without any of us having to look out for our partner or make excuses for why they didn't show up or had to duck out early.

And in case this hasn't been love letter enough to my new friendship, consider this: early during the 2020 lockdowns, when both families were hunkering down outside the city, still avoiding contact with anyone outside our own nuclear foursomes, Ali got a bad case of COVID. Chris and I decided to have a little fun and try to lift her spirits. (We had another close friend with COVID at the same time, so we did this twice over.) He created a boom box out of cardboard and put an iPhone in it, and we drove over to Ali's house. I called George, found out which room she was holed up in, and stood in front of her window, in my long trench coat, and held the fake boom box in the air blasting Peter Gabriel's *In Your Eyes* in a full John Cusack *Say Anything* moment.

"Did you do that just to make me laugh?" Ali asked me.

The answer, duh, was of course.

"That," she said, "is friendship."

9

They Flew the Coop

ON BEING AN EMPTY NESTER

I n August 2021, I hit that parenting milestone that we spend eighteen years longing for but also dreading: I dropped my first child off at college.

Rowan always wanted to go to Wake Forest. My nieces went to school there, and every Thanksgiving and Christmas my girls would hear their cousins' stories about the friendships and the parties and look longingly at their photos of the campus and the dorms. To them, Wake Forest represented the quintessential college experience. I used to bring them to my own college reunions, at Princeton, and they were completely uninterested—they wanted the college life they saw in the movies, with Greek life and keggers and athletics. The whole rah-rah vibe. Rowan, especially, wanted to be farther away from home. I just wanted her to go to a school she was excited about, and I couldn't have been prouder of her when she got into Wake Forest.

In many ways, you raise your kids for this moment—you want to equip them to be independent adults, to launch them so that they know how to take care of themselves and pursue their dreams and be functioning adults in the world, ones who know how to interact with others without a parent interjecting with reminders to say please and thank you and make eye contact; to lock the door at night; to get to class on time in the morning. It's exactly what's supposed to happen. And not just to us! You see it in the animal kingdom: male elephants stay with their family unit until about sixteen years of age, and then leave the herd to go out on their own. Mama birds push their little ones out of the nest so they can learn to fly. In each case it's a survival mechanism, a way to set your child up to make it, even thrive, on their own in the big bad world. But just because it's necessary doesn't make it easy.

When we dropped Rowan off at school for the first time, the four of us drove together from New York to North Carolina. Chris had the foresight to know I might be emotional on the way home and that I wouldn't want to be crying publicly on an airplane, so we made the nine-hour trek by car. That weekend, we did all the typical freshman orientation activities: carried her luggage to her room and helped her unpack, made multiple trips to Target, took her out to a nice dinner, toured the campus, met new classmates, attended welcoming ceremonies. In some ways, it felt like the parents were going to college too—we went to parties, played beer pong, and pretended we were kids again . . . and then it all came to a crashing halt. On our last day in North Carolina, I tried everything I could to stay a bit longer. *Maybe we should make one last trip to Target! Do you need a different shower caddy?* Rowan, too, tried to find extra assignments to keep us together a bit longer: folding clothes, organizing drawers, refolding clothes, reorganizing drawers. We were both dreading the inevitable, but at around 3:00 p.m., standing in her dorm room—which was now personalized with photos of Rowan and her friends, posters of New York, and inspirational quotes (YOU'RE DOING GREAT BITCH), and a purple neon *R* next to her lofted twin bed—it became clear that the time had come. Chris, Rowan, Grier, and I walked to the parking lot near the dorm. The three of us hugged Rowan individually and then as a group, and got in our car to head home.

As Chris pulled away from campus, I watched as my waving daughter got smaller and smaller in the rearview mirror, and when I say I wept . . . dear God did I weep. I am not exaggerating. I was choking on my sobs, barely able to breathe. I ended up doing needlepoint while listening to an audiobook in my earbuds the entire ride home so that there was no space to contend with any emotions. (Therapy much?) "The saddest drive away from anywhere" is how I described it in the subsequent Instagram post, and to this day that feels accurate. But what stunned me was how much I absolutely did not expect it. I'd been so busy making sure Rowan had everything she needed and planning the logistics that I never thought much about how I'd feel when we parted. If anything, I figured I'd be excited for her above all else, so I was more shocked than anybody when we pulled away and the tears started falling and didn't stop. I was gutted! I wanted to immediately turn the car around, pack her dorm back up, and begin looking for colleges within a two-block radius of our home. Or even better, apply to get my teaching license for homeschooling! Kappa Kappa Henchy sounded great to me. I was proud, for sure, and happy for her, too, but in the moment? Mostly I was devastated and couldn't believe this day had arrived. When they're babies, you just can't imagine them ever not being babies. I felt desperate.

Having Rowan away at school was the first time our family had been separated. Sure, I would travel for a movie or other work from time to time, but it was always pretty brief, and they were all together waiting for me to return. I would FaceTime my family every day. I always knew what they were up to, even if I was filming on the other side of the country or the world. Same when Chris was away for work. But my kids never went to sleepaway camp. We took our vacations as a family. Grier's boyfriend went away to camp every summer, and when he first told her that he'd be leaving for four weeks, she was so confused. "Why?" she said.

"What do you mean, 'why'?" he asked. "It's camp."

But my girls never wanted to leave. Grier's boyfriend turned to me out of nowhere one day. "Mrs. Henchy," he said (the boys have decided on their own to call me Mrs. Henchy—to me that's my mother-in-law, but Mrs. Shields would have felt like my step-mother or something from a fan), "your girls really like being around you and your husband."

"Well, we have fun," I said.

"That's really special," he said with his sweet little smile.

When the time came for Rowan to return for sophomore year, I didn't even go along for the drive. "I can't watch you in the rearview mirror again," I said. "Just tell me when you're coming back to visit, and I'll focus on that." (That time I posted a video on Instagram—me standing on my porch in tears, *again*, after having said goodbye for the second time. Of everything I posted that year, that reel got the most engagement—clearly, it's not just me who struggles with these departure days.)

For her junior year, Rowan went abroad to study in Florence. She'd been a little bit homesick during her earliest days at Wake, but that passed quickly. In Europe, on the other hand, everything felt so foreign, literally and figuratively, that for a while she was really out of her comfort zone. She wanted to come home within the first couple weeks, and I could relate. When I went to college, I was desperate to come home. And I was in New Jersey, only one state away from my mom! It wasn't exactly being in Europe. My very first semester, I cried and cried and cried. I would go home on Friday after my last class and stay for the weekend and drive back Monday. Every week. I also made my mother drive out every Wednesday to take me out to dinner. I was so isolated—not because people were mean but because they were trying to give me my privacy. Eventually I made some friends and joined a comedy group and found my footing, but it took a while. And when Rowan was homesick while abroad, there was definitely a part of me that took some solace in it. *Awwww, she's homesick for me!* But healthy mom mode kicked in quickly and I was able to speak from experience. "You'll always regret it if you come home," I said. "This is a short period of time—only a semester—so you need to dive in and find your people and your place." A part of me absolutely wanted to send her a ticket to New York and have her jump on the next flight so all four of us could pile into our king-size bed with the dog and watch a movie, but there's a difference, in parenting more than anything, between what you selfishly might be dying to do and what you know you should do, for them. I didn't want her to miss out on this experience. But I didn't entirely hate that she felt a pull to come home, either. (It might very well have been the familiarity and comfort of her college that she missed, but no harm in projecting the missing onto myself. I am sure it was at least a little bit of both. Right??)

When we got Tuzi, our dog, we had a dog trainer come to the house. Tuzi is a little Houdini, and when she first got to our home she would take any opportunity to make an escape. If she's a bolter, put a leash on her, the dog trainer told me. Make it a thin, light one, and have her drag it around all day so she knows she's tethered. I don't hate that Rowan has that sense of tetheredness, too. I do want her to remember where she came from, and to feel the pull to return home from time to time. And yet I also want her to thrive on her own. Nothing is such a mixed bag of emotions as becoming an empty nester. You want them to love home, but you want them to be okay on their own. You want them to be independent, and yet there's some delight when they still need you. You want to let them be their own person, and yet you worry about them more than ever. There's a whole new set of threats to fret over when the kids go off to college—the partying, the sex (that you are not aware of), the crime rate on campus, whatever. Rowan has type 1 diabetes, so I'm wondering if she has the necessary amount of insulin and updated medical equipment at any given time. Now she wears a monitor, and I get the alerts sent to my phone, but we've made a deal that I only call her when she goes too low. I resist calling when the blood glucose number goes high and I just keep checking that it begins trending downward.

Being this connected is a blessing and a curse. When she was abroad, I crossed my fingers that she remembered her passport or knew how to book the tickets when she would visit different countries, and then I'd stare at the phone, waiting to hear that she made it to her destination safely or that she didn't run into any problems or get targeted for being an American tourist. It's hard not to be petrified all the time. It's like they leave home but they still come first, because you're constantly preoccupied with the fear that they're going to die. (It sounds melodramatic, I know, except if you're a mom reading this, you know of what I speak.) Plus, the simple truth is that you just miss them being near more than you could ever have imagined. At least that was my experience. And you can't run and pick them up if things go wrong—you just have to hope and pray that you've given them the tools they need.

My mother didn't give me the tools I needed. She controlled me so much, in every possible way, that when I went to college and had to navigate the world on my own, I was in shock. I was like an open wound. Totally vulnerable. I wanted something different for my girls, and I tried to arm them with the ability to trust their instincts and keep their wits about them and be prepared and self-assured and self-protective. My mother made it her job to protect me, and while I did have a sense of always being tended to, loved, and watched over (which can feel really nice as a kid), she also did me a disservice, because for so long I had no clue about how to actually protect myself or live on my own.

My girls have a lot of skills I never did. And I'm so glad for that—I would be devastated if I felt I'd repeated my mother's mistakes in that regard. I have always aimed to re-create all the joy and fun my mom introduced into my life, without all the trauma. It makes me proud to see how competent my girls are, and though missing them injects some melancholy into this stage, there's excitement and joy, too, because you're not just launching your kids. You're launching yourself as well. Once Rowan was gone I still had one more year before this nest was completely empty, and yet those same gut-wrenching tears and dread at leaving my last baby in a foreign place soon bubbled to the surface. But there is also a type of renewal, or at least a kind of revival, embedded in these rites of passage. Sending your kids to college and going back to a house that's just you, or you and a partner, is the beginning of a whole new phase of life. One that comes with the same fear and uncertainty as your kids are grappling with, but also the same exhilaration and freedom.

When Rowan left home I was already considering building a business for women in midlife, but watching my kids leave the house really highlighted for me how important it is to look at this next phase of my life and closely consider what I want it to look like. Because suddenly, I can do anything. It's not just the freedom of not having a kid at home, which is pretty major in itself. No longer do I need to worry about doing pickup, or about taking a job that will force me to travel. I also don't have to worry about accidentally contradicting myself or opening the apps on my phone too slowly or inadvertently making a hypocritical decision or simply *breathing* wrong. My daughters, they watched me like a hawk, and there's some comfort in being able to move around the house without the unforgiving eyes of teenagers in every room. To revel in a lazy Sunday or say, *Yes, I think I will enjoy another cocktail, thank you.* But there's also a freedom of discovery in this period. With all that time I once spent catering to my girls, I can now cater to myself. I started taking dance classes for the first time in ages, and I can't think of any word to describe it other than joyous (albeit slightly more painful than I remember). We learn the samba and the west coast swing and the Lindy, and by the end of the hour my brain and my body are so tired, but it's that good, satisfying tired. There's a ninety-year-old lady who dresses impeccably with hair sprayed perfectly in place and this adorable little old man and people of every shape and size. You line up and dance with whoever is across from you and then you move down the line and pair up with the next person. Is anyone there going to be a professional dancer? No, definitely not. But there's so much happiness in that room! And it's not that my kids were explicitly preventing me from dancing before they left, but I just didn't have the brain space to look up the classes and get there and commit to it weekly. But now, with the girls gone, I can fill in all the space that was freed up by not having to keep track of high school sports schedules and social engagements and school calendars and fill it with activities that are fun for me, and only me.

Now, to be totally fair, Chris has always been a very hands-on dad and committed to watching the girls' various sports. Regretfully, I did miss some of their games and I can count the meals I've actually cooked for them over the years on barely two hands. We had a nanny who helped me navigate all of it, but I was constantly ping-ponging between each kid and all their activities and their life schedules. I'd run home from a job to tuck them in and then return to set or have them brought to the theater on matinee days. No matter how busy my life was, they were always my main focus. With no kids in the house, time feels different.

When Rowan left, it fundamentally changed the dynamic of our household. But I wasn't an empty nester just yet. There was comfort in still having Grier home, even if she was already an independent young woman who would be the first to tell you that she could handle herself on her own and didn't really need her parents anymore. Chris used to drive her to school in the mornings until her boyfriend started to give her a ride. And so it goes.

As I prepared for Grier's departure, I fell into a trap that I should have seen coming. When a household has one child gone and the other gearing up to leave, I've noticed a parent can go one of two ways: either they fully embrace their kid and hold them tight, glomming on and being clingy because they can sense a departure coming, or they begin to distance themselves as a protective measure. I occasionally fell into that latter bucket, and I had to make it a point to keep myself in check, not putting up a wall when what I needed was to soak up the time together. But it's hard when you can sense the inevitability of them leaving. I was dreading it so much that I tried to get ahead of it. It's like a breakup. You know it's going to be gut-wrenching, so you try to nip it in the bud.

Because Grier is very much my child, she took the same approach with me. One night, we were in a typical mother-daughter fight—she was suddenly mad at me for who-knows-what, and I was just staring, mouth agape, trying to figure out what was going on, when she yelled, "And I'm leaving and you don't even care!"

Ah, there it is, I thought. *Now I know what we're dealing with.*

I used to have a godmother who would come visit me every

year, and we would have a great three days together until, the day before she had to leave, she would start picking fights. She always had to leave mad. I finally said to her, "Is this easier for you than being sad? Is that what's going on?" The very last time I saw her, I put her in a cab while she was giving me the silent treatment. "You're going to cry all the way to the airport, aren't you?" I asked. She simply rolled up the window and drove away. It was too painful for her to have to say goodbye, and that was the last time I ever saw her alive. As Grier's turn to leave home came closer, I realized she was doing a similar thing. She was being harder on me because she knew she had to individuate, and the easiest way to do so was to find any reason she could to hate me. I got it. I didn't like it, but I understood it.

In one of our precollege arguments, Grier was annoyed with me because she felt I was trying to insert myself into a decision that wasn't about me. It's possible she was right. But it's also hard to change that tendency when, for eighteen years, your opinion was the most important.

"I hear you," I told her, "but you need to try to hear me, too. For years and years I told you when to go to sleep and what to wear and what to say and how to speak and how not to speak. I told you what to eat and where to be and how to be! Now you're becoming an adult, and you're discovering your own self, and that's great, but you have to allow me an adjustment period." It almost feels like a bait and switch. For two decades, this has been the life I've known, and then virtually overnight, it is altered dramatically. I definitely had a moment of, *I worked so hard and it just flew by!* But you can't do it any differently—even if you've savored the moments, it will feel like the rug has been pulled out from under you. But that's life as a woman. Every stage brings change and readjustment. There is certainly some relief that comes with your kids needing less from you (parenting teenagers is hard!), but it's also really sad and lonely in its way. It's like the first time your kid has a serious discussion with a friend and you're within earshot, so you try to jump in only to be met with "Never mind, Mom, you wouldn't get it." *What?! Wait just a second, missy. All I have ever done is gotten it. I've helped you through every piece of friend drama and conflict!* Or, God forbid, when they forget to give you a kiss goodbye as they leave with their friends to go to a party. It all just makes you ache.

When it was Grier's turn to leave, I had the added concerns of not only living in a house that was entirely empty of daughters but also the fear that I would lose closeness with her. Rowan is the type to call home a lot, and I knew that. Grier's more inclined to put up that protective wall. Plus, since she would also be attending Wake Forest, I knew she might just go straight to Rowan rather than call me when she wanted a dose of home.

Clearly, both my girls have become independent women. As a mother, you can know, intellectually, that it's going to happen, and it can be exactly what you want to happen, but living it and witnessing it feels different. For so long, I was the center of their world. If they fell down and skinned their knee, they came to me. I wasn't the kind of mom who freaked out with worry, but I would clean it off and put on the Band-Aid. I had a part to play. When they leave it's like you're suddenly demoted to the understudy—you're waiting in the wings and you're watching from the side thinking, *I'm good at this part! Let me go on!*

The first time I went to visit Rowan at college, once she was settled and had made good friends, I remember standing off to the side, observing her with this group of girls I'd never met. But these girls *knew* my daughter. They understood her and they saw her. They were laughing with her and crying with her and having smart discussions with her and I had nothing to do with it. It was a wake-up call, but also as sure a sign as any that she was going to be okay. I had this feeling of, *Well, I guess we actually did a decent job of raising these girls to be self-sufficient and independent.* But that was immediately followed by, *WAIT, WHAT?! I take it all back! I want a do-over! I want them back!* Parenting—it can really mess with your head.

Whoever came up with the phrase "empty nest" knew what they were talking about. So much of what we do as parents is about creating a home and rituals and making memories. You create a safe environment and nurture these baby birds, and the truth is: even when they stop relying on you, and sometimes even on your very body, you are never entirely done parenting and caring for them. But suddenly you look around and there really is an emptiness. But empty isn't necessarily a negative. Empty means there is space. There's opportunity for fulfillment from something new. From dance class! Or time with friends! Or a new career! Or doing nothing!

A friend of mine called recently after sending her younger son off to his freshman year. "I am loving my boys being at college!" she said. "But what does that say about me as a mother?" She saw quickly what took me a bit to realize: if parenting is done right, the kids leave with confidence because they know you're always there loving them, and available to them . . . and in the meantime, you can have some fun of your own!

Any notion that we are bad parents if we aren't desperate to be with our kids 24/7 is misguided, if not a trap to make moms feel guilty. This *should* be an exciting time. I had hot tears when my girls left, but then I was faced with the opportunity to get to know myself again, and to reintroduce myself to the various personal relationships that had for so long taken a back seat to my kids. This new stage can be full of promise and potential.

When I finally started to embrace it, I felt as wide-eyed as Rowan looked when she arrived on the Wake Forest campus that first time. My new life was starting, too! Now I could set out to discover my likes and dislikes, to decide what's important to me and what doesn't matter anymore, because most of those preferences have changed since I last took inventory, probably two decades ago. In fact, one of the reasons I approached my career the way I did, passing on opportunities that would take me away from my family for too long, was so that I could enjoy this time of life without regret. I have seen so many actresses who seemed so sad in their later years—their kids were gone and they suddenly wished they'd spent more time with them back when they had the chance. Now, I'm not saying they made a bad choice, and I probably wasn't being offered the same roles they were, so the pull to work away from home was not as deep. It's certainly not for me to wear a martyr hat or to judge. I would never criticize another actress's decision to take the work when it's offered, or shit on any mother's decision to work at any stage. When my kids were little I *did* work, just in a different, and lighter, capacity. But I know myself, and I know I would have beaten myself up if I'd missed their younger stages, so I made the conscious choice not to put myself up for jobs in the same way I had in the past. Now, if Scorsese had called me to film in some distant location while my kids were little, would I have packed us all up and gotten them educated in a yurt for a year? Gladly! In a heartbeat! But it was made very clear to my agents that during that period of my kids' lives, it would take something really incredible and irresistible to get me to travel wherever the work took me. And as it turned out, the Scorseses of the world were not knocking on my door, so I was never faced with the dilemma.

t's difficult for me to describe the sacrifices I made as hard, because as much as work has always been a source of fulfillment for me, it has never given me the same pure joy that my family did. I wanted to take advantage of that joy while it was accessible to me. But it was something I had to fight for. I had to resist putting myself out there in the ways necessary to stay in the game. I understand what a privilege it was that working less was even an option—Chris was working, which helped as a buffer, but plenty of women have no choice but to keep earning an income, whether they want to or not. But for me, stepping away from my career was hard in its own right. I'd literally never not been working. Still, I knew I would never forgive myself if I didn't stay strong. And I made those choices in part so that I could now harness a new kind of joy, the kind that comes from feeling like it has been earned. A joy that comes from the freedom to focus on oneself. That joy is very real, too.

Consider this headline that I came across on CNN: HAVING KIDS MAKES YOU HAPPIER—ONCE THEY'VE MOVED OUT. Most research supports the idea that child-free adults are happier than parents, but a 2019 study[1] found that this is not always the case. In fact, this study, which used data from a survey of fifty-five thousand people aged fifty and older, found that empty nesters experience more joy and fewer depressive symptoms, in part, the authors reasoned, because children transition from dependents to social contacts. (Research also shows that, in general, age does relate to a parent's happiness. According to one study, while parents younger than thirty are less happy than their child-free counterparts, parents in their forties and beyond see an increase in happiness alongside the size of their families.) I am still Rowan's mom, that's for sure—you're never really done with parenting—but it's also true that we have a friendship now that we never could have had when she lived at home. We talk on the phone and gossip and she asks me for advice about stuff, but she also asks me about my days and my own life. There's a bestselling parenting book called *All Joy and No Fun*, but as they get older and sometimes even hang out with you by choice, kids *are* kind of fun. I used to say "I'm not your friend, I'm your mother" when they complained that I wasn't being cool. But now there's something really wonderful about hanging out with them as friends. We enjoy each other. It's fun to have a glass of wine with your kid! But being without them? That can be fun, too.

I wasn't entirely alone of course. Chris and I moved in together when we got engaged, and lived together for more than two years before Rowan arrived on the scene. Now we were back to just the two of us, and that was its own adjustment. Our life was so different before we had the kids—we lived in L.A., I was doing a sitcom, we dated and got married and were pretty fixated on our common goal of starting a family. Now we had to find a new normal (more on that in a bit) but I was also faced with more solitude than ever before. Sure, I wasn't completely alone, but when you go from four in a home down to two, there's a lot more alone time. It's just math.

When I was younger, being alone made me panic. It felt like wasted time. I wholeheartedly believed I should be filling every moment with conversation or fulfilling an obligation or checking a box or just *growing* somehow. But these days, I love solitude. I had to learn how to appreciate it, but now being alone doesn't equate to loneliness. For so many years, every step of the way, someone has needed something from me—my children or my jobs or my husband or my family. There's this *Family Guy* scene where baby Stewie stands next to his mom Lois's bed saying, "mom mom mom mama mama mommy mommy mom ma ma" and she finally screams "What?!?!?" and he just says, "Hi." That's parenting in a nutshell. Suffice it to say, once I had kids, finding time alone was a form of freedom.

Loneliness in middle age can be truly dangerous. It's bad for your health, and as plenty of research has shown, it's a predictor of an early demise. But solitude is a very different thing. It's an intentional choice, one that allows you time for self-reflection and to enjoy your own company. Loneliness, on the other hand, usually involves a longing for something different. For company or companionship. Research shows that adults benefit more from solitude as we age because we develop more control over our time, as well as better cognitive and emotional skills to help us use that time more constructively. One study found that adults ages thirty to fifty-five in particular pointed to competence (specifically building new skills), self-growth, and self-care as the benefits of solitude. This group, and even more so elder adults, were also interested in the autonomy that comes with solitude, described as "a space in which they could feel self-reliant and connect with themselves, free from the pressure of others."[2] I do think it's an earned appreciation—I'm just more comfortable these days in my own skin and sitting with myself and spending time doing something I enjoy, alone. It's like riding in a car with someone and not feeling compelled to speak. Feeling comfortable enough with myself that I can be alone and doing something that gives me joy is such a relief, because there's no pressure to keep a conversation going and no worries about holding anybody up or doing something their way. There's no performance anxiety or judgment, which can be the defining features of interactions for so much of a woman's life.

My favorite solitary activities are going to the theater or sitting at a restaurant with a good book. When I did *The Addams Family* on Broadway, I took myself to see the play *Jerusalem*, alone, after rehearsal one day. This is a three-plus-hour, two-intermission performance. I loved it so much I saw it four more times, and never once let anyone go with me. But until Rowan went to Florence, my solo activities had been limited to a few hours at a time, and always close to home. I went to visit her abroad around Thanksgiving and spent the days solo while she was in school. At fifty-eight, it was my first time being alone in a foreign city.

I have spent my whole life traveling the world, but I was always with my mother or a bodyguard or an assistant or Chris or on a movie set with a handler of some kind. This trip, there was no assistant director telling me where to go, no PR person instructing me on talking points, no assistant reminding me that I have another Zoom in ten minutes, not even a family member with an obligatory agenda. I have journeyed, but always with at least a girlfriend. To be roaming around Italy, with no one aware of exactly where I was, it was a bit unsettling for me. But also exhilarating! I wore a baseball cap and sunglasses, which meant I blended in with most American tourists, and that presented another form of freedom. I wandered into cafés and talked to store clerks and sat at the base of the Duomo with a Peroni, gazing up at the stunning architecture. I got lost and spent a lot of time on Google Maps, but it felt like a long-overdue rite of passage. I'm coming up on sixty, but I'm still growing up and trying new things and learning about myself, and while I don't know that I will make a habit of solo travel, it's good to know that I can enjoy my own company even for long stretches of time.

Sometimes, if I'm feeling especially sad about my girls being gone, or especially excited about having my house to myself, friends will remind me that they don't always leave for long. Especially in New York City, with rents as high as they are. I wouldn't be surprised if my girls both move back in eventually, as they try to find their way in the world. But even when they come back, they don't *really* come back. It's not the same as it was before, and it never will be. And I think that means we've done our jobs right, as parents. I joke that I am planning on my girls and me becoming like *Grey Gardens*. What's wrong with that? They'll feed me cat food and wear all my clothes again and it'll be great!

But until then I'm trying to accept the mixed emotions—for every moment of sadness when I feel like I'm missing a limb, there's a moment of joy when I remember I can go to a dance class without checking the school schedule. And when things get especially dark, I just remind myself: without them here, I've found all my favorite articles of clothing that miraculously disappeared over the years. I feel like I have a brand-new wardrobe.

10

Sex and the Middle-Aged Woman

MEN, MARRIAGE, AND THE MALE GAZE

I arrived late to my friend-of-a-friend's soiree, but not too late to miss the tour of the fancy prewar, beautifully renovated brownstone in Midtown. The owner was a newly divorced man with two children. The house included a walk-through wine cellar, complete with corking station. My husband loves red wine, and because I could see some amazing vintage bottles with labels I knew my husband would swoon over, I sought out the owner to ask about his wine. I figured that anybody with a collection as extensive as this one would surely have reason to be proud, and would probably enjoy discussing it. As he displayed the different vintages, I asked a couple of questions about which years he likes to buy and why, and we ended up in a discussion about how wines improve with age. He explained that he likes to buy bottles to commemorate significant years in his life. "I'm a '72 vintage, a great year," he quipped, referencing the year he was born.

Attempting some levity, I responded with: "Well, I'm a '65. An even older vintage! I may have you beat."

I was about to follow up with a question about how a '65 Châteauneuf-du-Pape drank, but as soon as I referenced my age this guy's face dropped. It was as if by admitting the year I was born, I had suddenly shattered some secretly held expectations.

In a split, unsettling second, I could see this man trying to reconcile 1980s Brooke Shields with the mental math that a '65 vintage made me—*gasp*—fifty-eight. "Oh man," he said. "You really shouldn't have told me that."

I thought he was trying to make a joke, but this was such an obvious knee-jerk reaction that his words came out more like a scolding.

"Why, because it makes *you* feel old?" I asked.

"Well yes, there's that . . ." he said.

And . . . what? I wanted to ask, but I was kind of in shock, and true to form, I resisted being rude. I was in his home after all. (Old habits die hard!) Only moments before, this man had been borderline flirty and happy to pontificate about grapes and regions and vineyards and rare bottles at auction. I had wanted to ask him if he could suggest a not-too-crazy bottle of wine I might be able to buy for my husband for our anniversary. But I never got around to it, because the moment my actual age was brought up, his demeanor and the entire, previously comfortable exchange morphed. The fact that I, someone who he presumably remembers best as a pinup from his childhood, could be close to sixty, ruined something fundamental for him. It made him feel ancient and maybe irrelevant (and maybe even somehow disappointed in me?) to hear I could have aged all these decades. The implication was that I should keep my "vintage" a secret or be ashamed that I have the audacity to be almost sixty, because that meant I could no longer be the dream girl or have sex appeal. Well, news flash, I'm not on this planet for the sole purpose of making you feel virile. Just then my husband arrived and I deftly passed the torch by saying, "Oh, here he is now, my husband, who absolutely loves red wine. I'll leave you two to discuss."

The way I interact with men and the way they respond to me—whether it's the men I know and love, or those I've never met—has changed a lot as I've matured. Being famous makes a difference, of course. I am often less overlooked by the men I meet because they typically know who I am. As it did with the guy in the wine cellar, talking to me in some way feeds their ego. At least until they know how ancient I've become! But on the flip side, if someone doesn't realize that I'm Brooke Shields, I'm invisible. It's like there is no middle ground. And when I'm with my daughters? Forget about it. The men's stares are blatant, and you'd think I was not in the room. It's at these moments that I am caught between feeling protective of my beautiful, fresh-faced baby girls and ready to lunge at any guy who even glances their way, and feeling like I somehow have lost my own long-standing value or appeal.

It all bothers me less than it once did, but no one likes to feel invisible. But I've also hit an age where I know my self-worth and don't need the male gaze to help me decipher whether I'm valuable. I'm also, thankfully, happily married and not out there on the prowl. I have friends who have separated from their husbands after decades together (is it a coincidence that this timing aligns with sending their kids to college? I think not), and they're having a tough time out in the dating world. Still, even if I'm not looking for romance, the way men receive me is noteworthy, because the patriarchy is real. When men stop noticing you, it's a pretty good indicator of how the world at large is going to treat you.

Of course, men treating women as less than—wanting to keep us small in order to take up as much space as they can—is not limited to a specific age range. I've had to deal with insecure men my entire life. To be clear, I've known and worked with wonderful men, many of them, and these guys respect women in general and respect themselves and know that those two things are not mutually exclusive. (I married two men who respect the women in their lives tremendously.) But when, for example, you're an actress who is first on the call sheet in a rom-com, playing opposite a handsome man, you will get a front-row seat to what the male ego can look like.

For a long time, I was primed to expect cattiness from women. In *Pretty Baby*, for example, my most difficult relationship among the cast was with Susan Sarandon, who played my mother, because I don't think she appreciated the eleven-year-old on set getting so much attention. (We have since worked together and remain friends to this day, but at the time, it was tough, for both of us, I'm sure.) But as my career progressed and I had the opportunity to star in more films, my female costars were almost never an issue. Women generally support each other and are just happy when we get to be in a movie with more than one strong female character. It's the men who've usually been the difficult ones. If I'm the lead in a romantic film and it's my character's story, my male costar is often noticeably rude to me. He'll talk down to me and say things like "You'll want to stand on your mark," as if this is my first foray into filmmaking. During one shoot, the director actually eliminated the big kiss moment because the actor was being such an asshole to me. (I find this is less often the case with A-list actors because they are confident in their standing. If a man isn't secure in his success, that's when he takes his insecurity out on his scene partner.) I'm pretty friendly on any given set and I like to connect with the guys working behind the camera. On more than one occasion I've had teamsters say to me, "You want him to walk home with a limp? We can handle it Friday when we're done filming. We don't like the way he treats you." They're probably joking, and I haven't accepted the offer to find out for sure, but I certainly appreciate the sentiment.

The truth is, for a long time, I never thought of myself as a feminist. I think I had a misguided understanding of what feminism was, and I thought that being a feminist meant you had to be angry at men. I realize now, of course, that we can love men and still insist that they acknowledge they are a big part of the problem. I like to say that when it comes to at least some men at this stage of my life, I'm not angry, I'm just disappointed. I think we could be met with a little more celebration when we reach these years. What I've seen happen instead is that as we grow more comfortable with ourselves and more confident, men grow more threatened. They simply don't know how to adjust. All this change upsets the balance that they've become comfortable with. Maybe the woman in their life simply feels less inclined to check in with and accommodate them because she has less to prove. Maybe she's returning to work so she's no longer the stay-at-home mom, always putting her family's needs first. Basically, women are changing both themselves and their lives while men want everything to stay the same. And who can blame them? Their lives have been set up, pretty deliberately, to work for them. This new discrepancy between the sexes can be cause for a bit of a reckoning.

Chris and I have been together for twenty-six years. People are always shocked to hear I've been with the same man for more than two decades. They don't expect it of a Hollywood relationship. Of course, I had a starter marriage. One of the reasons I married Andre was that I liked being in a relationship with someone more famous than I was. After a lifetime of always being the focus, it was a relief to be able to slink into the background a bit. He was a gallant guy, too, and I loved that. People would always ask him, "Why do you get up when she leaves the room?" And he did. If I rose out of a chair, so did he. He would say, "I want her to know that I'm waiting for her to come back." He was a gentleman like that. And I liked all that traditional stuff. It also felt good to be treated as something a little bit precious. All while he was the center of attention. Less pressure.

When Chris and I first met, in 1999 at the gym on the Warner Bros. lot, I was still married to Andre. We became friendly because we'd see each other at that gym from time to time—I was working on *Suddenly Susan*, he was writing for a show on the lot—but we didn't start to date until the following year, after I'd gotten divorced. When Chris and I first got together, I was broken. My marriage had ended, my best friend had just died, and my father had been diagnosed with cancer. I felt like Chris swooped in and folded me into his arms. That he saved me. Some might consider it diminishing to admit that, but the truth is, I loved it. I've always been a sucker for romance, and I liked the whole knight-in-shining-armor approach.

When you get engaged, you're signing up for the bliss—the wedding planning and the big celebration and the honeymoon. It's potential as far as the eye can see. The reality includes all that, hopefully, but also the strain of family and money and work and life. I had a lot of preconceived notions back then about what marriage should look like, both in general and in Hollywood. When it came to work, I was tough on Chris toward the beginning of our marriage, because I wanted to star in the TV shows and movies he was writing and producing. I wanted to be his muse! He worked with Will Ferrell on *Land of the Lost* and *The Campaign* and *The Other Guys*, and as far as I knew most Hollywood producers seemed to be casting their wives in their films. Obviously, there is so much that goes into casting a successful movie but because I was married to Chris I assumed I would be his leading lady on- and off-screen. And in fact, early on, we did have some opportunities to work together, and it was always a joy. People on set were amazed at how well we communicated and our lack of conflict. Chris would even suggest tweaks to my lines, many of which were better than the original script. We were a great team.

Those experiences subsided pretty quickly, though, and I became frustrated. It was by no means why I fell in love with him, but subconsciously, my actress brain had created an elaborate dream sequence in which we became a Hollywood power couple. I knew I wasn't being fair, and I was putting too much pressure on him and our relationship. Ultimately, I told him that unless he wrote a part specifically for me, I had to be taken off the consideration list, because I couldn't audition for him. The awkwardness of it would make me freak out and my ego wouldn't be able to handle the rejection. Not to mention that as an actress, we are not privy to the producers' opinions or reactions behind closed doors. Think of the position I was putting him in, being on the other side of the door as producers or casting agents or executives were possibly saying negative things about his wife.

People often wonder how our marriage lasted this long—that might be our secret. The truth is that there's enough work to go around, and our marriage and our soon-to-be family needed to have its own starring role.

In the decades since, Chris and I have gotten to know almost everything about each other. The other day he shared a story I'd never heard before and you'd think he'd divulged who shot JFK. *You've never told me that! We've been together twenty-six years!* I don't even remember what it was except that it was something trivial. But it shocked and excited me to hear him recount a story I'd never heard. You lose the mystery after all this time, which eliminates a bit of the excitement. Plus, behaviors that you might once have found endearing because you were blinded by love might now just seem, well, annoying. Chris and I know each other so well at this point that I can anticipate his mood by the cadence of his footsteps on the stairs or by the tone of his voice when he answers the phone. And despite the time that has passed, I think he's very much the same guy today that I married twenty-three years ago. Sometimes, that's where things get hard. In that time, I've changed exponentially. I've grown more confident and self-assured. (You might remember the research I mentioned earlier, about how women's confidence improves over time while men's stays relatively steady.) I'll stick up for myself more, even in the little moments. Chris loves to tease me. When we were courting, I thought it was cute. He's a really funny guy—he's a comedy writer for god's sakes—and I was impressed with his wit and was fine with being the butt of the joke. In fact, both Chris *and* the girls like to make fun of me. It's the plight of the mother, I think. Let's tease mom, who doesn't drive well or know how to bake or is a neurotic actress! Meanwhile, guess who they're calling in the middle of the night when she's on set in Phuket because they can't find the poster board they need to bring to school for a presentation the next day? I try to be good-natured about the barbs, but sometimes the same old jokes just aren't that funny anymore. To be picked on, even if it's all "in good fun," makes me feel bad and inept, and with age has come an ability to advocate for myself even with my family, rather than playing along lest they call me too sensitive.

One of the recurring themes of the teasing is my cooking, because I don't do it. I own this fact—I even have a series on my Instagram called "Brooke Don't Cook." But there was a time when I loved cooking with Chris. He knows what he's doing in the kitchen, and I enjoyed it when he taught me. I wasn't an especially quick study, I guess, because eventually either he got impatient or even more set in his ways of executing things. These days he generally won't let me near so much as a cutting board. But recently, we were having friends over and I was helping out in the kitchen. I was toasting pine nuts, and I stepped away from the stovetop to get something from the fridge at the exact wrong moment. When I returned to the pan, the pine nuts were brown and burned. I redid them, and it was no big deal, but I knew enough to say, "Do me a favor, when our guests arrive, can you not open with a joke about how I ruined the pine nuts?" Being forward like that used to be terrifying to me because I hated confrontation. Now, gritting my teeth and pretending to be amused just doesn't work for me. Standing up for myself and saying "That's unacceptable to me now" has been empowering. It doesn't have to come off like a confrontation or accusation. I've learned that if I can say something to the effect of "I need to express something to you: this is how I took what you said and I need to understand why you said it," and if I can say it calmly (and usually after the fact, when the hostility in the room has died down), it doesn't put him on the defensive as much. And to Chris's credit, I'll see him think about what I've said and try to do it differently next time. It's not always graceful but I acknowledge the good intentions. Not all my friends have been so lucky with their partners—I should count it as a win.

I've also grown more independent, as a person in general, but also as a wife. I love Chris very much, but I don't need him the way I once did. I don't need saving anymore, and I think being the saver was as satisfying for him as being saved was for me. It was part of his currency. To take those "manly" opportunities away from some guys can feel emasculating. I also don't need Chris in the purely biological sense, because I've had my kids. All that change puts us in a very different place now than when we got married. It forces us to be intentional about our relationship. To make our marriage work, I have to want him in my life, because I don't need him in the same way. And I've said as much to him, because I think you have to be honest in order to get on the same page. "I'm not using you," I said to him once our girls were grown, "and yet a huge part of your purpose in my life has been satisfied. Now we need to get back to the things that made us fall in love and remember why we chose each other in the first place."

If you've raised children with someone, it's tough to get back to the dynamic you had before you built a family. Remembering how to spend time together without the kids around, to talk without planning child-rearing logistics, takes work. It's hard enough, in fact, that plenty of couples can't do it. There's a new term, "gray divorce," which refers to the increasing divorce rate for older couples who have been married for a long time. Overall, the divorce rate in the United States has been on the decline. According to the CDC, the divorce rate dropped from 9.7 divorces per one thousand women in 2011 to 6.9 divorces per one thousand women in 2021. The one group for whom divorce is on the rise? Adults aged fifty and older. In fact, in 1990 only 8.7 percent of all divorces in the United States were of partners fifty and older. By 2019, that same age bracket accounted for 36 percent of divorces.[1] That's a huge increase! (The divorce rate for couples over sixty-five has actually tripled—one in ten people getting divorced these days is sixty-five or older.) Researchers point to a handful of reasons for this: the population as a whole is aging and staying healthier longer. Because of that, even at fifty-five or sixty-five you can see that you have plenty of time left—maybe you don't want to spend it in an unhappy marriage. (Good for you!) Couples are also marrying later, so if they are getting divorced, they're likely doing that later, too. At the same time, studies also show that empty nest status can have a positive effect on marital closeness. As the authors of one such study explained, "As the chronic demands and challenges of parenting children diminish for couples who are living in the empty nest, they may have more time, energy, and resources to cope with other stresses and to improve or maintain their relationship quality, particularly compared to couples living with children at home."[2] Both sides—the increased divorces and increased closeness—make sense. When you're in the throes of parenting, you really are *in it*. It's hard to focus on the marriage, whether you want out or you want to feel more bonded.

Relationship satisfaction hits a low point around age forty.[3] It's an age when most of us are still working but also potentially raising kids and also dealing with elderly parents. And the kid piece matters—findings show that parents tend to be more unhappy with their relationships than couples without children. Once you can come up for air, you might look at the situation around you and start to consider what you actually want. On the one hand, you might think, *We've had a good run.* On the other hand, there's a lot of comfort in being with someone you know so well and who knows you, and the idea of starting over might sound like torture. And, of course, you might just really love whoever it is sleeping next to you at night.

Having grown children—and thus having to refocus on ourselves and reexamine our relationship—has not been without its difficulties for Chris and me. There was definitely a moment of "What are we going to do now?" You sort of need to reintroduce yourselves to each other, which is a little bit scary because it's not going to be how it was when you fell in love the first time. As I've mentioned, we've changed, and so have our circumstances. First of all, we both work largely from home. If I'm not on a movie set or traveling for a speaking engagement, I'm doing business for Commence from my home office while he's writing in his workspace one floor up. It doesn't offer a lot of opportunity to miss each other. We don't really talk about our days because we're right there, watching them unfold. We're not the couple that will sit around and talk politics (I would ask if those couples exist, but they do, and they are Ali and George), and we know so much about each other that the discovery phase is long gone.

We also have different ideas of how we want to spend our free time. We used to work out together, but since my femur injury that's been less of an option. A big part of Chris's social existence—the thing he looks forward to every day—is dinner. He loves to go out to eat and sit at the bar and chat with friends or bartenders. I don't really want to be eating at nine—I'd rather go to bed early with a book or a TV show and get up to exercise in the morning—but if I want to spend time with my husband, that's the time to do it. I weigh things differently now. What am I going to remember at the end, that I took another 8:00 a.m. spin class or that I had a great conversation with my partner? Which is why sometimes, despite wanting to be in my pajamas, I throw on a pair of heels, meet him at one of our local haunts, and order his namesake "Hencherita": a margarita without the sugar.

One thing Chris and I absolutely have in common—always have and always will—is that we both like to win. We're competitive people. It's a blessing and a curse. As we've tried to find activities to engage in together in this grown(ish)-children phase, we dabbled in pickleball. We played together a few times, but he's so intent on winning that he does these spin serves that he knows I can't return, so now I refuse to play with him. Competition is fun; constantly feeling like a loser isn't. During the pandemic he taught me how to play dominoes, though of course when I started winning he attributed it, at least at first, to beginner's luck. I like dominoes fine, but my game of choice is backgammon. I have a group of gay male friends in Southampton with whom I'll sit on the beach all day and play cribbage and backgammon. Last summer, I taught Chris to play after much convincing. My dad played with me when I was very young, but he never really taught me any strategy. (Dad was more of a "throw the kid in the pool and they'll figure it out" kind of a guy.) My father was quite intimidating—in backgammon and in life—but that should be its own book. Playing with Chris, however, was really fun, at least in the beginning, in part because I usually won. Well, that turned out to be a short-lived joy. Soon I started to notice him practicing! Instead of playing with me he'd be on his iPad playing some sort of solitaire backgammon, and now when we play, I am often the loser. I think I may need to move him to cribbage and see how long that lasts.

At the end of one summer Chris asked me, "Do you need to get a gay husband? You seem to have much more fun with them than you do me." I explained that my other "husbands" and I are just not competitive in the same way. Plus, we revel in the same experiences, whether it's spending hours on the beach or antique hunting all day together, and we are actually relaxed and revived by doing so. Chris gets bored with most vacation activities very quickly. Then, one week, we were in a funk. We just weren't in sync, which always makes me feel panicky. I get worried it means we're drifting apart—that it's the beginning of the end. That week, every exchange between us had an edge to it. We couldn't talk without bickering. When one of those moments turned into a full-fledged argument, I wanted to talk it out and he didn't—same old, same old—and we were at an impasse. He left the house to run an errand, and I was at home stewing and unsuccessfully trying to get work done when he called and said, "Do you want to grab the backgammon set and come sit with me while I get a coffee? We could play a couple games?" It was an olive branch, and it worked. We didn't have a big talk but it got us back on the same page, or at least on pages closer together. A marriage counselor might say we need to repair rather than just distract (I don't know for sure; while I love therapy, Chris . . . not so much), but

I appreciated his gesture. I ran into an acquaintance a couple weeks later who said, "A friend and I saw you and your husband playing backgammon together outside the coffee shop. We both thought it was the sweetest thing." I didn't point out we were playing because we still weren't talking.

These days, backgammon at a nearby French bistro has become something we do semiregularly, or at least when we know we need a reset. I don't know if Chris enjoys it as much as I do, but he does it for me, and so I go to late-night dinners for him. It's important to me, because I know that if I start living too independently from him, I'll get really good at it, and that's dangerous. The spouse relationship is so primary to me—the idea is to get old with this person, that he's who I'll be left with, so I want us to still like each other.

It's impossible to talk about men and women and aging and relationships without talking about sex. *Are you having it? How much? Do you even still like it? Does it hurt?*

I had a fervent sex drive when I was young, but I never felt like I could step into that appetite in the way I wanted to. I lost my virginity to my college boyfriend and first love when I was twenty-two. I waited that long because I had the weight of the world on me. Not just figuratively. The whole world really was watching! And even once we started sleeping together, I never really let loose. I was so in love with him. He was so beautiful and I so wish I could look back and think, *Oh wow, that was a wild time. We just went at it!* It was perfectly set up to have been that carefree, can't-take-your-hands-off-each-other young love, but my mother, the fans, and especially the public had such a hold on me. I stupidly and guiltily confided in my mother after I lost my virginity, and once she knew, whenever she'd get drunk she'd shame me about it. "I know it's just physical between you two," she'd sneer. My connection with my boyfriend was a personal affront to her, because having a man in my life in such a real way meant that she was losing me. Oh, how I wish I'd just let the lust take over! But regrettably I was never able to do that.

And now here I am, more than thirty-five years later, sometimes pretending I'm asleep when I know Chris is in the mood. And that has nothing to do with Chris—he's hot! He's been working out at a boxing gym recently, and he looks incredible. Women are acting differently toward him, and I can see it. And he loves it! I can see that, too. At the same time, I'm going through all the bodily shit that comes with aging as a woman even in the best of times—the thinning hair and the peach fuzz and the brand-new belly fat and vaginal dryness and the diminishing sex drive—and in my natural state I feel less appealing to him than I ever did before. It makes you think, *Oh, this is how it happens.* Men can still have children, so they're just as valuable to younger women even in this age. But women can't at my age, and a huge part of our appeal has been our ability to bear offspring. To be able to give birth and carry on a man's legacy is a powerful magnet. Once that's gone, a huge part of our currency to men is gone, too. And mostly my response to that is a big "get over yourself," except then, when I want to attract Chris, it's on me to find ways to be sexy, and I resent that, too. I resent getting to a place where I'm expected to do more work to keep a man's attention! Haven't I worked hard enough? And yet I do feel the pressure to keep it up, to maintain his gaze, lest he find someone "better" (translation, in this case: younger).

But back to pretending I'm asleep. It's not great, I know. I was talking to a doctor recently who inquired about my sex life and I explained to her that I have no desire and I'm fine with it. Turned out, she was not fine with it. I'm hardly unusual—reduced sex drive starts for most women in their late forties and fifties.[4] While men also see a general decrease in their libido, women are two to three times more likely to experience a decrease in sex drive. My doctor didn't particularly care about these statistics. Just because it's common doesn't mean it's good. I ended up on the receiving end of a lecture about how important sex is to a relationship, how couples need it to connect, how it can ward off depression and boost immunity and reduce stress, and how it improves communication between partners. Not having sex, she said, can erode a lot of what brought a couple together in the first place. It may not be the same as it was in your younger years, but it can still be good! Pleasure is important, for both parties. And because of all that, she said, I need to get my hormones in balance.

I know these are all valid points. But, on a personal level, I'm in a place where sex can be painful. Thanks again, Dr. Malpractice, for the bonus surgery years ago. (I shared the story with my gynecologist, who told me that his little "tightening gift" was a huge contributing factor to my pain. Jesus!) For me to fully enjoy sex at this point, I need my lotions and potions, the right sleepwear (maybe calling it sleepwear is contributing to the problem), my special pillow, and maybe a tequila so I can relax. Again, Chris is not at all the problem. Did I mention that he's HOT? All the more so now than he was on our honeymoon. Listen, there's nothing wrong with using whatever you need! Whatever it takes. My doctor told me I should start taking testosterone—*Sure you might get a few more whiskers, but that's what tweezers are for*—but I haven't gotten there yet. For now, I'm counting on the old "the more you have it, the more you'll enjoy it" approach.

Low sex drive isn't the case for all women, of course. And even just believing that sex is important can make a difference. When women between the ages of forty and sixty-five place greater importance on sex, they are more likely to stay sexually active as they age.[5] And here's what I definitely know about the importance of sex: when Chris and I are in a fight, while there's nothing I want to do less than have sex, if we do, he assumes that's the end and everything is fine. He literally becomes less angry. I don't want to resolve conflict by sleeping together, but I think that's important to understand. I'm not saying sex should be used as a weapon, and consent is, of course, always a prerequisite. I guess I just believe that sex is always going to be powerful, so let's use that power on our own terms.

Here's what I want the men in my life to know: I love you! I do! We love our partners and our male friends and male colleagues. But we don't want to love them at our own expense. I don't want to love them more than I love myself. I had nothing to gain from sitting back while being chastised by the guy with the wine cellar except being deemed "likable" by someone who clearly had his own issues with aging to resolve. I could have laughed off his comment—*You really shouldn't have told me that*—but I'm tired of getting my hand slapped for no reason. Especially when the thing I've done "wrong" is to simply have the audacity to survive and exist and get older and admit it.

I'm not saying I always feel the need to correct someone in these situations. Honestly, if deferring a bit to a man's ego can benefit me in some way, so be it. But there are plenty of times when there's no reason for me to sit back and bat my eyelashes while men talk down to me. If age has gifted me anything, it's the ability to see both scenarios, and the wisdom to know the difference.

11

The Parent Trap

ON THE CHANGING
RELATIONSHIP WITH YOUR KIDS

After my getaway to Florence to visit Rowan on her semester abroad, the two of us traveled to London, where we met Chris and Grier for Thanksgiving. We were in the apartments connected to the Ham Yard Hotel near Soho for the holiday, and one morning I walked by Grier's room, where her suitcase was open on her bed, overflowing with my belongings. A Dior sweater, Prada shoes, a Chanel bag. All the stuff with a recognizable label was currently in her possession. I didn't say anything to her, but inside I was seething. *These are my nicest clothes! I don't even wear them! How dare she take my things without asking, and pack them like it's no big deal!*

I was more annoyed than I should have been. Sure, a child shouldn't take a parent's stuff without asking, but this was certainly not the first time. That Grier had helped herself to my clothes wasn't really what irked me. They look better on her anyway. But there was something deeper going on. It was her nonchalance about wearing such nice things—she knew these were not everyday outfits but my nicest designer duds—that I found so triggering. Was I jealous of her freedom? How is this young person able to not only appreciate but also revel in all this quality apparel? She can exist joyfully in garments I still don't allow myself to wear, even though I own them. I'm willing to spend the money, but whenever I buy something nice or expensive, I "save it." For what, I'm not sure. I keep my designer clothes and accessories in the closet, in perfect condition, waiting for some special occasion when they "deserve" to be worn. It doesn't make a lot of sense, because most special occasions call for something fancier than jeans or a sweater, which means my nicest versions of those items usually go untouched for months or years at a time, and often go out of style before I've even enjoyed wearing them. Now, I've never been a trendy starlet wearing only the hottest looks—mostly because they're too expensive to justify owning, and if I wait they most likely go on sale in the not-too-distant future. I love going to places like Century 21 and the Woodbury Commons outlets. But I digress . . .

I mentioned the incident with Grier on the phone to my therapist. "And she's walking around in a Christian Dior sweater as if it's no big deal! She's wearing my best clothes, things that I spent my money on but never wear myself!"

"Why don't you?" my therapist asked. Typical. Shouldn't she have been joining me in my outrage?

I didn't have an answer. I'm still trying to unpack what it was in my upbringing that made me feel unworthy of enjoying the fancy (read: expensive) items I own. It certainly had something to do with my parents—my dad wanted me to be a "regular" kid and barely acknowledged my fame, my career in movies, or my subsequent paychecks. Wearing nice clothes meant I was buying into the notoriety that he didn't approve of. As an adult, that has translated to me eschewing fancy clothes in favor of more casual and affordable outfits. It's an effort to appear more down-to-earth. My mother, on the other hand, believed she was the ultimate consumer. She subscribed to a belief in quantity over quality. She always preferred to buy ten low-quality department store cashmere sweaters rather than investing in one beautiful one. "Why don't you spend the money and get one nice piece and just take good care of it?" I'd ask her.

"Why buy one when you can have ten!" she'd say.

I vowed that when I got older I would never buy the ten shitty sweaters but instead invest in the one quality one. (Mom did, however, buy seven properties around the country by the time I was in my late twenties. . . . Maybe it was a Depression-era kid thing.)

I worked so hard and so consistently for decades without ever really spending my earnings on myself that as I got older, spending money became a kind of rebellion for me. My mom would say things like, "If we do this project, we can get a car," or "If we get that campaign, we can move into a house." My connection to finances was directly tied to the quality of our living situation.

As I got older and started buying designer pieces, I never had guilt or felt bad about spending my hard-earned money. So why then did I squirrel them away, too afraid of ruining them, saving them for some unknown future occasion? It's so strange to me that the joy seems to be in the buying more than in the wearing. I often take my pieces out of the closet and look at them but inevitably choose a less-expensive item. Kind of nutty if I'm being really honest! After I turned fifty I promised myself that I was going to use my nice things, but it's been easier with silverware and china, or perfume and makeup. I've even managed to start wearing my nice shoes more often. But wardrobe-wise, it's still a challenge.

The combination of my two parents' teachings gave me the

sense that while I might be able to afford nice things, I couldn't just wear them around like I was "fancy" or a big deal. What's the opposite of a sense of entitlement? That's what I had.

It turns out, when you do your therapy session over the phone in a glass-paned office nook at the foot of the stairs to your daughters' rooms, there's a good chance the other people in that home will overhear your conversation. My therapist was still on the line when Grier stormed into the room and started throwing my clothes at me.

"I gotta go," I said quickly as I hung up the phone.

"You're talking to your therapist about me!" Grier yelled through tears. "You're acting like I'm a brat and a label whore!"

"I'm not! Not at all," I said. "I'm actually trying to figure out what's going on with *me*, and why I'm having such a strong reaction. You did something that's totally normal for a teenage girl to do. And you have good taste!" I explained to Grier that I realized I'm embarrassed to wear my nice things because I want to be perceived as "regular." Maybe I'm even a little bit jealous of her, because she can enjoy luxurious clothes without it bringing up complicated feelings of guilt or discomfort or self-consciousness. And she really does treasure them and take care of them and return it all, so this really is just my shit.

"Wear your stuff!" she yelled at me. "I went into your closet and you know your Hermès bags? They're covered in dust! What are you saving them for? You work hard for your money. You've earned it. And you're going to die one day! I hope not soon, but it's going to happen, and then what? You'll die with a closet full of unused clothes!"

I started laughing and crying all at once.

"What's so funny?" Grier said.

"There will come a time, if you have children, when they'll start teaching you things instead of the other way around," I said. "You spend eighteen years schooling your kids and molding them and one day, out of nowhere, one of them says something so insightful, so smart, so revelatory, that it knocks you over."

For me, this was that moment. Everything Grier was saying was true. I *had* worked hard for everything I owned. I *was* going to die one day, whether I enjoyed my fancy handbags or not.

"You are *Brooke Shields*, Mom," Grier said. Usually my kids don't acknowledge or care much about who I am other than their mother, but I saw her point. "When people say 'Brooke Shields is so down-to-earth,' what they are probably really saying is that you don't have style. That you look like a mess!"

Okay, that last part seemed a little extreme. I have never actually read that people think I look sloppy or unkempt. In fact, I have often gotten "wore it better," but I saved that little tidbit to myself. I heard her loud and clear, and I got the point of her rant. I couldn't even be offended because I was so busy wondering when she got so mature. When did my baby turn into an adult? And a really freaking smart one at that! These days I've even started wearing all the apparel that had been collecting dust in my closet, because she got through to me. It was as if all my years of undermining my successes and saving my stuff because I worried about what my mom would say just melted away. I felt like I had been given some sort of reprieve.

Now that I don't worry so much about how I'm being perceived, I actually enjoy my nice things.

It is a momentous shift when you start learning from your kids. And I'm not talking about picking up random facts about the Revolutionary War that your second grader learned in social studies, or the weird new math they teach in schools. Why does no one "carry the one" anymore? I don't know. But when your kids impart wisdom, or help you see yourself in a new light, or help you understand the world a little bit better, that can blow your mind. It's just one of the major ways the parent-child relationship changes in this era, which I'm discovering in real time. It's something I am particularly in awe of and enjoying tremendously.

When I was still in pigtails, I did an interview with talk show host Tom Snyder. "What do you want to be when you grow up?" he asked me.

"Well, I want to be a mother," I said. "I mean, I want to continue acting but I also would like to be a mother, because I love kids."

Say what you want about my relationship with my mom (everyone else already has), but we had an incredible bond, and I knew since I was little that I wanted a version of that relationship with kids of my own. To my parents' great credit, I always went to nonprofessional high schools. There are plenty of performing arts schools in New York City, but forgoing them helped me understand that there was a world out there beyond the entertainment business. Even at a young age, I knew I didn't want my existence controlled entirely by an industry I wasn't sure I had a lot of respect for. Or that had any respect for me for that matter. It treats people badly and thrives on insecurity and fear. On its best days, the world of entertainment fosters creativity, and when you're able to exercise that creativity it's a brilliant business, because it's about art. But when you are reliant on the industry—for recognition or to affirm your value or even just for financial security—you are at its mercy. I somehow understood this at some level, and I knew I was too sensitive to not have a fulfilling life of my own to fall back on. I also knew that if I had a family to fight for and a place where I felt entirely at home, it would distance me just enough from the industry to stay sane.

From the time my girls were babies, I had a sense of what kind of mother I wanted to be. I tried to speak to them like they were little people, worthy of having opinions and being respected. I didn't condescend or speak to them like they were lesser citizens. I wanted them to feel listened to and not judged. Don't get me wrong, I was a stickler for manners, and they knew they weren't the boss. My mom always billed herself as someone who was nonjudgmental—she really hung her hat on that—but that's not how she came across to me. I always felt like I was going to be in trouble for something, or I would be wrong, and I was often waiting for the other shoe to drop. This is a consequence of being raised by an alcoholic, and I was always a little skittish and on edge. Work, even if I knew both the industry and public opinion to be fickle, felt stable in the sense that when you were on set, the space was contained and there were rules by which you had to abide. You and your schedule were always accounted for. That was freeing in a way. At home with my mom, on the other hand, I never knew what was going to happen. Plans would change at a moment's notice. So would moods.

I wanted to protect my own kids from living with feelings of instability, uncertainty, or fear, so I built in routine and ritual wherever I could. I encouraged them to be outspoken and opinionated rather than timid. At the very least I urged them to express their opinions when they had them. "How did that make you feel?" was a constant refrain, or "Why do you think you reacted that way?" when they admitted to doing something they shouldn't have. I wanted them to know that nothing was off-limits, that we could talk about anything. That didn't mean there weren't consequences, but we'd discuss why they acted a certain way. I was always proud to say that when it came to that age-old "You better [insert parental instruction here] by the time I count to three," I rarely if ever got past "TWOOOO. . . ." And if they did get in trouble, I always explained why. I tried not to introduce "because I said so" into my parenting lexicon, as tempting and easy as it would be.

Obviously, my relationship with my mother was complicated. So much so that it's the subject of its own book, but it's impossible to reflect on my parenting approach, and how my relationship with my girls has evolved, without thinking about all the ways my connection to my own mother changed over time. My whole life I went to her for absolutely everything. Yes, I feared being judged or reprimanded. Yes, I was guilt-ridden whenever I thought my behavior would disappoint her. And yet the pull to her was so strong. A magnetic field surrounded her, and even when I knew better, I was always pulled back in. Love is a very strong motivator, and there was no love lost between us, ever.

There's footage of my mom and me in the *Pretty Baby* documentary—I'm learning to dive and my mother is sitting poolside, giving me feedback. You see me pop out of the water and swim over to her and the first words out of my mouth are "What am I doing wrong?" She's directing me to "think out, not down, and think all the way across to the other end of the pool," and showing me with her hands from the comfort of her lounge chair, where she is fully clothed in a lovely pink dress. Only in rewatching the documentary did it dawn on me . . . she didn't even know how to swim! She was never taught, but I followed her coaching as if she were Katie Ledecky. That was our relationship in a nutshell. She was the expert, even when she wasn't, and I assumed that however I was doing something, I could be doing it better. To me, she was the arbiter of all things Brookie.

The one thing I did not consult my mother about was parenting. It truly saddens me that my girls didn't grow up knowing my parents. My dad died three weeks before Rowan was born, and my mom was already in decline by the time the kids were no longer babies. But even when they were babies, I learned very quickly that beyond raising me, she couldn't handle children. I wanted her to be the sweet little old granny (I should have known better) or the kooky brash fun grandma who spoiled them rotten (more likely), but instead she stood off to the side, not sure what to make of these children or of this new relationship of which she was supposed to be a part. The girls were alien to her—they were an extension of me and yet had nothing, really, to do with her, and something about that didn't compute. It was as if she wasn't even blood related, which she obviously was. The girls didn't respond to my mother the way I did as a kid—they weren't deferential or in awe of her, and she couldn't control them the way she did me—and I don't think she knew what to do with that. She wasn't jealous of them, exactly, but there was a notion of, *Who are these strangers taking up your time and your life and who have somehow replaced me? And why don't they, too, love me unconditionally?* (There must be whole chapters written on this type of reaction in a book I imagine is called *The Narcissist's Almanac*.) I think my dad would have gotten a kick out of my kids. They would have been innately respectful of him because of his size and manner and voice. He was a six-foot-seven man who really was larger than life. He also wouldn't have been threatened by them, and I'm not sure I can say the same for my mother. It never occurred to me that she would feel that way, but maybe it should have.

Rowan and Grier are very different people and have been practically opposites since they were kids. They both love me a lot, like any kid loves their mother, and I like to believe it's in a healthy way. They see my flaws and they get mad at me and they tease me, but they also stick up for me, and I think they respect me and want my input. Of course, all this while also finding me as annoying or embarrassing as any young adult might. When Grier was little, around four or five, she would get angry and say to me, "Mama, you are everything that is wrong with my life!" And then, five minutes later, she would adopt a very serious tone and say in her adorable staccato cadence: "You know, Mama? Every time I say something mean to you, I wish I did not say it but I cannot stop it before it comes out of my lips."

I may not have been the traditional mom in the 1950s housewife sense—not cooking or cleaning or doting on the girls every morning and night—but I raised kids in New York City in the early 2000s. June Cleaver is not who they were seeing anywhere, really. In fact, when Grier got mad at me her senior year of high school for not being a "normal" mom it wasn't that I didn't have cookies and milk waiting for her when she arrived home from school. It was that I wasn't tough enough on her. Not tough enough! And I gave her too much trust. Who knew there was such a thing? "My friends' moms are making them crazy and asking if they did their essays yet and are their applications ready, and you're just . . . not!" As I reminded Grier, I don't breathe down her neck because she's the most organized *person* I know, let alone the most organized teenager. Plus, she was a hard worker who asked a lot of herself. I didn't think it would be right to push more on her. And yet! You know what they say, if it's not one thing, it's your mother.

I wasn't a helicopter parent, hovering around and dictating my kids' every move. But like most moms, I was the family CEO—I scheduled the doctor's appointments and planned the playdates and made the lunches. But I was discreet. I made sure they were working hard in school and had incredible manners but I never had to hound them. I was also never the alarmist mom who ran to her fallen child howling "Oh my God are you hurt? Tell Mama, were you pushed? Who did this to you? Are you okay?!" My kids (especially Grier) would tumble a lot and always had bruises on their legs. Once I heard Grier nonchalantly tell another mom who was commenting on her bruises (bitch), "Yeah, I fall down a lot." Whenever they'd hit the ground I'd calmly help them up and brush them off, checking for blood and then doing some distracting dramatic gesture, yelling "A perfect ten! Yippee!" Mine are New York City kids, so they got more independent as time went on and probably more independent than their suburban counterparts would be at the same age. I'm not sure exactly what it is about city kids, maybe it's that they can get places on their own without needing to drive, or that some take the subway to school on their own by the time they're fourteen. Those teen years are funny—in many ways, they want you out of their lives. They want to flex their grown-up muscles and experiment and get away with things. And yet they want you around at the same time—at arm's length, but available nonetheless—to be friends with their friends' parents and show up to the soccer games and go to the parents' nights. And, apparently, to micromanage the college applications.

Close, but not too close. Involved, but not too involved.

The height of my conflict with my girls coincided, perhaps not surprisingly, with the onset of menopause. Changes in hormones affect your mood, your body, your comfort level. It's not your fault, it's biology! But as far as the kids are concerned, it's your fault. I would get hot in a room and start peeling off layers and I'd catch the girls rolling their eyes at each other or stifling a laugh. If I was irritable, and roller-coaster hormones will make you irritable, I got a lecture. "Mom, you're impossible to live with," they'd say. Or, "You're heightening the anxious energy in the room." My mother changed the energy in every room she entered, but that just wasn't the way people talked back then. I, on the other hand, raised my kids to express their opinions without fear of judgment. Their opinions, it turned out, were basically "Mom's a pain in the ass." At least for a short but memorable time, I admit that was the case. They said it with such disdain, and during the height of those days it was all I could do not to lecture them on the physiological changes of the fifty-something female. Their time would come. (Of course, this timing was such that my girls were probably undergoing their own hormonal changes just as they mocked mine—hormonal changes that made *them* more irritable or impatient or, one might say, pains in the ass themselves. It was a perfect storm!) I do believe that if more people understood those physiological and biological shifts in mature women, maybe we wouldn't be blamed for so much. But my kids didn't understand, so now not only was I irritable thanks to the aforementioned hormone fluctuations but I was also irritable because the people I lived with blamed everything on me. There's only so long you can take that before you snap.

If postpartum depression was my unlucky consequence of being pregnant, these moments of rage were the aftermath of no longer being able to be pregnant. I'd reached the other side. Back then I wanted to jump out a window, now I wanted to push everybody else out.

I kid, I kid. Sort of.

I've mentioned this already, but the onset of my menopause coincided with the onset of my daughters' womanhood. When they were little I tried so hard to help them become strong and independent people—and as they grew older, I wanted to help them become strong and independent women. This was another area where I wanted to diverge from my mother's parenting approach. I didn't want to insert myself into my daughters' dating lives, but I did want to impart some advice that I wish someone had given me. And I wanted them to know they could discuss whatever they needed with me without being judged. Maybe this isn't so much the case for mothers with sons, I really don't know, but having daughters who were coming of age forced me to reexamine my past. I was such a good girl. I was always so measured. It's not a point of pride for me, quite honestly. I wish I had more of a past. More rebellion. More sex, safely. I've tried to encourage the girls to recognize this period of their lives as prime for experiencing and experimenting. I'm not bohemian about it, but I am realistic.

I've surprised myself a bit, because I find myself saying things to them that I never even thought of for myself until ten years ago. Things like "your pleasure is important, too." I don't want them to have any shame. Don't get me wrong, I don't want to hear too many details. (Remember when I said my kids were opposites? Well, Rowan tells me things that make me want to cover my ears, whereas Grier announced early on that "I will never discuss any of this with you, ever!") I want my young adults to enjoy this time—there's nothing like the early twenties—in a way that is healthy, and also a bit selfish. Don't wait until you're married, I say. That's my honest advice. That doesn't mean having sex isn't a big deal. In fact, it can be the biggest deal, so you want to make sure it's good but also safe. And only if and when you choose it. Sex matters in a relationship, but it's a two-way street. You want to make sure it's good for both parties. That it satisfies him isn't nearly enough.

When Andre and I were married, people would ask us how important we thought sex was to a marriage. "If it's good, it's the least important part," I would say. "If it's bad, it can affect the whole thing." I'm still pretty prudish about sex talk even to my therapist because it's hard-coded in my cells to be ashamed, but I don't want that for my daughters. I want them to find someone they care about and trust and I want them to have fun with that person. "Don't give it away freely," I'd say. "But if you're in a relationship that has mutual respect and admiration, celebrate that. I never had that when I was younger, and I really wish I did."

It's tricky, being honest with your kids about your past. When they're little, it doesn't feel entirely relevant. You can speak from experience without necessarily *sharing* your experience—you're simply an authority. Wear sunscreen. Be careful near the stove. Don't put anything in writing you wouldn't want shared publicly. Sure, you could share the story of the time you got that bad sunburn when you were eight, but your kids probably won't care all that much, and as far as they're concerned you didn't exist before they came along. You are not a person, you are simply their mother. But then they get older and life gets more complicated, and they might learn more from hearing about your messy past than listening to a lecture on how they should or should not behave. Still, deciding what to share and what to keep private can get messy in itself. Part of the reason I wanted to do the *Pretty Baby* documentary was that I had daughters. I felt a responsibility to help shine a light on the way we treat young women in our society. The best way to do that, I decided, was to be forthcoming and share the entirety of my experience. Where I was remiss, however, was that I forgot to be forthcoming with my kids before I was forthcoming with the world.

In the documentary, I opened up for the first time about a sexual assault I experienced at the hands of someone in Hollywood in my twenties. For so long I kept it secret—I felt guilty, and ashamed, and talking about it was too painful. I told the story in the documentary as part of a larger exploration of sexuality and agency and victimization. And as an example of my refusal to be a victim, in so many different areas of my life. It was only one short segment in a two-part film, and I didn't want it to become the main headline. Of course it inevitably did, which I guess was to be expected, but only for a short time. I have no regret about what I did or did not reveal in that film. What I regretted was only that I didn't tell my girls in advance. Grier left the movie screening halfway through the film, in tears, and that felt like an error in judgment on my part. "I can't believe someone hurt you like that. I will never be okay knowing this!" she said. I should have warned her. Rowan's reaction, on the other hand, was, "Young women need to see this, Mom." Grier has a tendency to want to bury her head in the sand about uncomfortable topics, whereas Rowan lets it all out and expects the same from others. Neither approach is ideal in the extreme. But knowing what to reveal of yourself and what to keep to yourself, especially as your kids transition into adulthood, is a hard needle to thread.

Rowan called me recently from Florence and asked, with great curiosity, if I've ever tried mushrooms. I haven't. When I was growing up in the 1970s and 1980s mushrooms were consumed very differently than they are today. People didn't know about microdosing back then (I hardly know about it now). When I thought of mushrooms I pictured someone sitting on a couch staring at their own fingers for hours at a time. I'm sure there are students at Wake Forest, like any university, who are experimenting with all kinds of substances. I certainly feel some pride that my girls feel comfortable talking to me about drugs and inquiring about my experience and presumably having my answers inform their decisions. I feel grateful, too, that I can be honest with them. If I'd had some epic mushroom trip, I would have told her. But then there's a part of me, when I get a call like that, that thinks, *What is happening? These are my babies! Why are we talking about mushrooms like we're all hip and enlightened? How did I get here?? And for god's sake don't try something for the first time in a foreign country when you have no idea where it's from!* I even kind of wished I had survived more escapades, so that I could answer my daughter from experience. After all, how can either of them put credence in what I tell them *not* to do when I have never even tried these things myself? But the truth is I was always too scared, and still am. Still, I try to treat my daughters like adults these days, because they are adults. They are my babies, but they are adults, and I want to be their ally. I want them to always trust me. (In the end, Rowan decided not to try the mushrooms, and added, "If I did, Mom, I'd want to do them with you anyway." I had to say, "Sure, so wait and refrain while you're there. We'll try it together." Thankfully the topic has not resurfaced since. Bullet dodged for good, I hope.)

There are aspects of having actual babies that I miss. Mostly the snuggles. When we got Tuzi, our dog, she helped fill that void a bit. I am one of those people who said I would never allow a pet to sleep in bed with me, and yet there she is every night, under my covers, with one part of her adorable puppy body always touching me. There is something so primal about a baby stretching their hands out to you and scooping them up, and that feeling that you're the only one they want in that moment. I don't get that entirely from a dog, but it's the closest thing at this point. Plus, clearly I'm desperate because I am so allergic to dogs that I have to keep a nebulizer by my bed. I even got her a sleep onesie that helps tame the shedding and dander that could potentially send me to the ER. But the comfort and companionship she provides makes me desperate to adjust to living with this pup. (Grier "borrowed" my Gucci loafers the other day and did not put them back in my room but left them on the kitchen table. You can imagine what I discovered the next day . . . leather confetti!)

There's this idea that once your kids leave the nest, you're less involved in their lives. This would make sense, since they don't live with you. But I don't feel less involved. I mean sure, I'm not as needed in the logistical parts, the mental load pieces, like signing them up for sports teams or filling their prescriptions. And what a joy that is! Those are necessary parts of parenting, but they aren't the fun parts.

Although my girls are entering their adulthood, I would still describe myself as highly involved in their lives. I FaceTime or talk to them basically every day. We take family vacations together. I know what classes they most enjoy or friends they're hanging out with or boys they're dating. Most summers I feel like we're running a boardinghouse and I love every moment of being with them and watching them with these friends, who they'll probably have forever. Chris and I support them financially. That's the way of the world these days. "Most parents are in fact highly involved in their grown children's lives [two new studies found], texting several times a week and offering advice and financial support. Yet in many ways, their relationships seem healthy and fulfilling," reads a *New York Times* article about the relationship between parents and their eighteen-to-thirty-four-year-old children.[1] A report from the Pew Research Center titled "Parents, Young Adult Children and the Transition to Adulthood" found that 77 percent of parents describe their relationship with their adult kids as excellent or very good, and 41 percent say those kids rely on them either a great deal or fair amount for emotional support.[2] And parents are actually enjoying their adult kids! "These parents, who are Gen X, are more willing to say, 'Hey, this is good, I like these people, they're interesting, they're fun to be with,'" Karen L. Fingerman, a professor who studies adult relationships with their families, told the *Times*. The kids are generally happy with the arrangement, too. Sixty-nine percent say they are satisfied with the level of their parents' involvement in their lives; 59 percent describe their relationship with their parents as excellent or very good.

My relationship with my girls has changed so much over the years. It's still changing. I continue to worry about them— that will never change—but I'm learning from them, too. They surprise me and delight me. I've always said that if I were their age, I'd want to be their friend. They make me laugh. Rowan worked during the summer of 2023 at *Good Morning America*, and one day they featured the interns in a segment about Barbie-related products. When the anchors got to Rowan, they asked her about the pink nail polish she was testing. "I feel like I've been transported . . . to the dreamhouse," she said with a serious tone and straight face. It was so quick and witty and so genuinely *her*. Grier has started modeling—she's signed on with Tommy Hilfiger—and her work ethic is already a marvel. She has also been the youth representative for the Hope for Depression Foundation for the past two years, speaking on the importance of being open about mental health. She is going to fare just fine in this crazy industry because she has a strong sense of herself.

That moment with Grier and my suitcase full of clothes felt like a milestone. Getting schooled by my own kid—I'm not sure I'll ever get used to that. Then there was the time I heard one of them say "I love you" to a male who wasn't their father—that was a milestone, too. Moments like this, the ones that catch me off guard and remind me how fast things are changing, keep coming in this stage. They come with mixed emotions—pride, surprise, melancholy—which is the hallmark of parenting a burgeoning adult. It's fun. It's exciting. It's new. But mostly it's an epic trip. No mushrooms necessary.

12

What Could Have Been

REDEFINING AMBITION

Sometimes I think about how my career might have been different. In the 1980s I auditioned for *Dangerous Liaisons*, the period drama that starred Michelle Pfeiffer, Glenn Close, John Malkovich, and Keanu Reeves. I wanted the role—badly. During casting, I was told that they were choosing between me and one other actress, a girl who was still relatively unknown. That newcomer was Uma Thurman.

Uma got the role, and the movie went on to be a box office success and a major awards contender. She was the right choice—I wasn't sexy enough or mature enough to give the character of Cécile de Volanges what Uma gave it. She was a perfect fit. And yet for a long time I held on to the idea that if only I'd gotten that movie, my acting career would have taken a different path. I would have been considered a more serious actress, or more respected roles would have come my way.

Back in the day, I never would have voiced these thoughts. My party lines were "everything is as it should be" or "what's meant to be will be." Acceptance acceptance acceptance. With age, however, I've come to realize that I was lying to myself a little bit. I didn't want to be a shoulda-woulda-coulda type. When something doesn't happen for you, you move on. But I'm human. I wondered.

For a long time, I thought being an ambitious actress meant being a specific kind of actress. One who won Oscars, who was considered a thespian. There were a handful of roles that Elisabeth Shue was offered over me, and each time I got the rejection I felt like a failure, because I put so much pressure on myself to be the "right" kind of performer. Plus, I knew I could do it—I could play tortured! I could be a dark villain! I could do so much more than anyone knew!

When I was in my early fifties, my godmother—who, as previously noted, had a tendency to behave horribly, neither godlike nor maternal—mentioned to me in passing that Sam Cohn, who was one of the most powerful agents in the 1970s and 1980s, had wanted to represent me when I was young. This was the first time I had heard anything about it! My God, I agonized, if I'd signed with him back then, it would have fundamentally changed the trajectory of my acting career. My mom would never have allowed it though, because if he was in, she would have been out. At age fifty I did feel a sense of satisfaction in knowing that this person, revered for his ability to spot the next big things and help mold their careers, saw my talent. I felt validated that someone with as keen an eye as his could see my potential. But mostly, hearing all those years later that I'd lost that opportunity made me think, *What the fuck good does that do me now?* My mom was my agent—she wanted to manage my career her way, and didn't want anyone else to get to me. Whether it was for protection or to keep me for herself, I can't really say, but she believed she knew best. I think about what my career would have looked like had I known, or if I'd had the guts to demand, a professional agent—any professional agent—earlier. Maybe I wouldn't have become someone they made a doll of or who had branded hair dryers (hundreds of which still sit in my garage). Perhaps I wouldn't have had to go to Japan to do a Nescafé commercial in the mid-1990s to keep our brownstone.

I used to look at Natalie Portman or Jennifer Lawrence and think, *Now these women have had exceptional careers*. They're talented, have strong heads on their shoulders, and are respected. Natalie filmed *Léon: The Professional* when she was twelve. In many ways it was her version of *Paper Moon* or *Pretty Baby*. *The Professional* came out in 1994, and the next thing Natalie did was play Anne Frank in *The Diary of a Young Girl* on Broadway in 1998. That's a smart move—one made with a keen eye toward being seen as a serious actress. I remember watching Natalie's star rise and admiring her performances, but also realizing that nobody did that in my era. My personal dream and deep-down goal was to do movies and only movies. It was all I could think about. Prior to Princeton, I was consistently making a movie a year and thought it would go on like that forever. But after four years out of the business, the offers came less often, and it was primarily from rejection that I ended up going into different mediums.

It's human nature to wonder about what could have been. To consider the roads not taken. Especially in midlife, as more so-called forks in the road are behind you, it can be hard to not wonder how your life might have played out differently. That doesn't mean you regret your choices, necessarily, but curiosity is normal. When it comes to career alternatives in particular, studies show that nearly half the working population considers "what could have been" on a regular basis.[1]

Even in moments when I've pondered different directions my professional life might have taken, I don't discount having had a pretty unbelievable career. If mine hadn't gone the way it did, with all the highs and lows that entailed, I might not be a "personality" who is offered various opportunities even when acting roles aren't flowing in. There is a commodity aspect to my celebrity that makes it possible for me probably (hopefully?) to be able to earn a living for the rest of my life. Plenty of actresses I truly respect—and even some who I have felt threatened by or envious of—don't have that same security. I'm quite aware that the ability to support a family in this business is a gift. Plus, I've been lucky enough to travel the world and meet amazing people. But as an ambitious actress and ambitious person, it took me a minute to resolve my definition of "success" with the way my story unfolded. Because sure, I've gotten to meet the most incredible people—I had a personal exchange with Princess Diana, I did a gig at Sea World with Lucille Ball, I starred in Bob Hope specials, I scored Elizabeth Taylor's shoes before she walked down the aisle in her wedding to Larry Fortensky so she wouldn't slip—but I haven't gotten to work alongside many of the greats. I don't get cast in ensembles, and rarely am I seen in serious movies opposite esteemed performers. I suspect it's distracting to have me in the cast list, because my fame is as much about my personal life as it is about my work. Being recognized in the way that I am has nullified my ability to blend in. Of course, I also understand that it's because of that recognition that I'm invited to do a show at The Carlyle or run for president of the Actors' Equity Association or—write a book! It's a mixed blessing.

For a long time, I didn't want to admit that I had these hang-ups. I barely acknowledged them to myself. And yet because of them, and because I had friends who were in fact highly esteemed thespians—people like Laura Linney and Laura Dern and Naomi Watts—I assumed that not getting the same acting respect meant I wasn't good enough. Not having a gold statue was absolutely a blow to my ego, and for so long it made me question my worth. But at some point along the way, my definition of ambition changed. I realized that I could chase some preconceived notion of what it meant to be a capital-*A* Actor, or I could work at being my best at what I'm really good at. For me, that was comedy.

When I was working on *Suddenly Susan*, something clicked. First of all, I was good! I just was. The role was challenging, but I emerged from season one really proud of this skill that I knew I had all along, dating back to the twenty-seven Bob Hope specials I did spanning about ten years, but which was never quite valued by the industry. I also understood the craft needed for good comedy. I could tell when something worked and when it didn't—and when it didn't, I could sense how to make it better. And comedy isn't easy. Executing a pratfall may not always garner the respect of a dramatic monologue, but comedy takes good timing and physicality and a willingness to let go and make an ass of yourself that not everyone can lean into. You have to be able to think on your feet and try new things on the fly. I really loved those years—I was going to work every day and had a spot on the lot with my name stenciled in spray paint on one of the concrete parking bumpers. I was doing work I excelled at. I felt settled, happy, and in my groove.

Discovering my knack for comedy was especially important because once I understood what made me uniquely talented as an actress, I could let go of this false sense of how my value was determined. I could more easily celebrate the variety of ways my actress friends shine. I can watch a talented friend like Naomi Watts be brilliant in a leading role and enjoy her performance without beating myself up or thinking I suck or wondering why I'm not talented enough to be hired for such impressive work.

It's exhausting! Hollywood specializes in pitting women against each other, but at some point, my attitude changed when I realized we can be in community without being in competition. We can be ambitious and also supportive. It's never either/or.

More than anything else, comedy requires instincts. You need to have a feel for how to play off someone else and when to go for a laugh and when to hang back. Even when you know what's in the script, or have been told what you *should* do, you have to be able to read the room.

As I honed my instincts in my day job, I got better at listening to my instincts more broadly. I'd spent my whole professional life living on a path of should—what my career *should* be, the kind of roles I *should* pursue—but on *Suddenly Susan* I learned to reject that notion. Comedy was my lane, and I wanted to stay in it. I liked where I lived.

I was nominated for two Golden Globes for *Suddenly Susan*, and I won a People's Choice Award for my performance in the show. I'd won four People's Choice Awards before that, but they'd all been for being a "favorite actress"—never for any project in particular. The win for *Suddenly Susan* made me proudest because it was for specific work I was consistently doing. And that work led to getting cast as Ruth Sherwood in *Wonderful Town* on Broadway, a show I headlined for more than six months. Doing Broadway, I feel compelled to point out, is not for the faint of heart. You're doing eight shows a week, and this was a physical one. It was epically difficult. But I survived, even if I eventually had to have six separate operations on my feet because of that show! I came out of that Broadway experience fully embracing the notion that going forward, I would own my talent on my terms.

One of the nice things about working in an industry for as long as I have is that I had the opportunity to try a lot of things and find my particular strength. It's not like I pivoted, exactly, but discovering my comedic muscles allowed me to create the career I wanted for myself. My ambition changed shape. I wanted to take on projects that best showcased my talents and challenged me in ways that felt motivating rather than miserable. Trying to contort myself to fit a certain type of career that would never work for me? It was an unforgiving exercise. But leaning into my silly side and going for the laugh? That was something I'd been doing even before I performed with the Triangle Club at Princeton. Once I established myself in sitcoms, I started to take more Broadway roles, which were sort of diabolical in what they demanded of me but still felt so good. Then I started dabbling with writing, because it was something I'd always wanted to do. This was all taking place in my late thirties and early forties, and I had other goals by then, too. To have kids. To find a partner. To build a life with those people who were separate from my career and could provide me more lasting joy. In midlife, I grew into myself in ways that were the result of decades of hard work and a commitment to learning and evolving.

I just don't buy into the idea that we're less ambitious as we age. The women I know in my peer group—my friends, my family, my colleagues—we are all pursuing something. Maybe we're less inclined to set a zillion goals, and to base those goals on what other people say we should do, but we're not wandering aimlessly or winding down either. It's true that I don't want to spend any more years of my one precious life chasing a measure of success that probably won't bring me any actual happiness should I achieve it. I could get an Oscar or an Emmy and put it on my bookshelf and stare at it every day, and of course I'd be proud, and probably make every human I ever met come look at it, take my photo holding it, and then see how heavy it really is before leaving my home. (I presented the Best Supporting Actress Oscar to Maggie Smith for *California Suite* in 1978 and was shocked how much that little golden statue weighed!) But I also imagine I'd get used to that view pretty quickly, and ultimately be the exact same person.

Historically, ambition has been defined as a drive that is specifically linked to career. But really, ambition is a desire to achieve a particular end. By those standards, I am absolutely as ambitious as I have ever been. I'm more laser-focused on my needs and desires and doing what it takes to fulfill them, because I'm better at knowing what will make me happy and what will not matter. I go after what I want. I still want to do comedy. I want to run my business. I want to have time for myself. I want to have time for my family. I want to do dramatic roles from time to time to flex a creative muscle. I actually feel more ambitious than ever, because I'm so clear on what I want. That clarity is a perk of aging. And I'm pretty clear on what I *don't* want to do also.

If you're reading this in your forties or fifties or sixties, this is probably true for you, too. What you want now is probably different from what you wanted in your twenties and thirties, but I bet it has less to do with seeking power or prestige and more to do with fulfillment. When you're young and just getting started in the working world, you may find you're trusted with very little. You go into work and just want to show what you can do—and it's a lot more than making the pot of coffee. (Research shows women are asked far more often to do the "office housework"—make the coffee, take the notes, plan the birthday parties.) You want more responsibilities because you want more independence. But as I've aged, if someone says "Want more responsibilities?" what I hear is "Want me to add more work to your already full plate?" Uh, no thanks. More challenges? Sure. Work that feels more impactful?

Absolutely. But women, especially mothers, in this country have endless responsibilities. And while extra responsibility might be a by-product of growing and learning and trying new things, or even going after a bigger paycheck (you work hard, get paid accordingly!), it's hard to imagine *more work* being the end goal.

In the 2017 anthology *Double Bind: Women on Ambition*, playwright Sarah Ruhl has an essay, "Letter to My Mother and Daughters on Ambition." In it, she writes to her mother: "I want, before you die, for you to feel at rest, to feel you've accomplished enough. To look around at this earth and say: It was good. And I wonder if that counts as mission or ambition. . . . Or does ambition only count as checking things off your own list and moving ever forward?"

While my professional ambition continues to endure in this age, Ruhl's idea that it can involve satisfaction and rest speaks to me. I covet rest. Quiet. I am fifty-nine and I think about the stereotype that this is the time we women sit on our asses and play mah-jongg all day. I laugh at the inaccuracy of it, but sometimes I also think, *That doesn't sound so bad!* But maybe I'll start with Rummikub. Would that it were so simple. I recently sat in the back of a car that was shuttling me from one day of meetings to the next, transferring my calendar from my phone to my planner just so I could have a clearer picture of how many crazy-long work days I had until I got a day of rest. It would be a full two weeks before things calmed down. Sitting on my ass, my ass.

Being ambitious is core to my identity. I've been working since I was eleven months old. I chose to go to college, while still working, because I wanted a traditional education alongside my very untraditional professional life. When opportunities came I said yes, emphatically, because working hard and striving for more was just reflexive to me, and it was reinforced by the work ethic encouraged by my mother. Once I was able to reframe ambition and understand it to mean something different from "go after the next thing, or the more prestigious thing," I began to take on projects I actually wanted to do and pass on those I didn't. When I focused on what I was doing, not where I was going, my work got better. And it felt better.

In September 2023, not long after I closed my show at The Carlyle, I did a weeklong run in the A. R. Gurney play *Love Letters* at the Irish Repertory Theater. It is without question one of the best plays I have ever done. In it, two characters—a man and a woman; I played opposite John Slattery—sit onstage and read letters they've sent each other, back and forth, for nearly fifty years. I've done *Love Letters* twice before, once in 1992 (at L.A.'s Canon Theatre) and again in 1993 (at the New Mexico Repertory Theatre), but I don't think I ever fully understood it until this run. It's such an emotional show, and so beautifully written. It starts off with the characters in second grade, but in the role, you don't behave like a second grader, all you do is say the words as written and you *are* a second grader. It's the kind of play that if you go with the intention to ACT!, you ruin it.

In this most recent run, I felt like I understood the character of Melissa Gardner in a way I never have before. I wasn't as old as the character is in her older years, but by the time I played in this last run, I had lived a lot more than I had when I first took on the part as a twenty-seven-year-old. I've had a greater depth of experiences. I've had love and loss, and I'm more open to tapping into those emotions, to feeling the character's sadness when it's called for and letting the material affect me. When I was younger, I lived in protection mode. I didn't want to feel all that much. That may have helped me in my personal life, but it didn't exactly help me grow as an actor.

This time around, every night, I would read the words (the actors sit with scripts in front of them) and I'd have to grip my chair to keep from getting choked up. I was present in a very different way. I'm aware of how affected that sounds, but as an actress it's key. It was as if I wasn't trying at all, let alone trying too hard. As a result, I felt strong and confident in my performance, and in my talent as a dramatic actor in a way I never have before. I was moved every single night, and so was the audience. It was one of the most satisfying acting experiences I've ever had.

There's this idea that "ambition" is a dirty word. That for women, it's unseemly. A 2022 survey from CNBC found that about half of women consider themselves "very ambitious," yet other research shows that ambitious women are perceived as "power hungry" rather than powerful.[2] (Ambitious men? Surprise! They are considered powerful.) I would say there are certainly some ambitious people, men *and* women, who seem to be driven solely by the need for power, and the need to control others. They are demanding and impolite and can't believe when the peons dare to talk to them. I've seen this on movie sets as well as in pitch rooms. Those people are, obviously, not very pleasant to be around, but they often do get what they want.

That kind of behavior just isn't in my DNA. There have been times, when parts didn't go my way, when I wondered if I would have been more successful if I was, well, kind of a bitch? But as I matured, I realized that ambition takes many forms. And it can change many times in a life. I could go after what I wanted without being rude or disrespectful. If you are self-assured enough, you can ask for what you want without apology, but without attitude either. Once I learned that, I got better at pursuing work I wanted to do. I stopped crossing my fingers and hoping the right project would come along, and instead decided to ask for things. To manifest my ambitions. Like that role on *Nightcap*—I reached out to Ali directly, and thank God I did. By her own admission, it never occurred to her that I'd be interested. But in being ambitious, not only did I get to dig into a juicy and fun and sort of psycho part, but—bonus!—I made a best friend.

In 2022, I took part in the season nine finale of *Impractical Jokers*. In it, I hosted my own dating show—*Brooke of Love*—in front of a live audience. When one of the jokers, who "won" the dating show, said his new suitor wasn't his type, I laid into him. It was the most fun I've had in a long time! So instead of saying "thanks so much" and going on my merry way, I said, "I'd love to work with you guys again." And not just to be polite . . . because I really wanted to work with them again! Now we're in discussions to develop an idea to pitch to a network. It takes so much effort to get anything greenlit in Hollywood these days, but they heard me and came to me with an even bigger project. Whether or not it gets made or goes anywhere is beside the point. What matters is that I put myself out there, self-advocated, and, at the very least, made some new fans in people I respect. Look at me, making things happen!

Here's the deal: I'm never going to retire. First of all, I have a life to maintain. One that I've set up, and that I love, but it comes with college tuitions and mortgages and costs that I need to cover. But also, and this is a biggie, I love my work. I like being creative and trying new things and making people laugh and working with other actors. I'd love to do another sitcom. The work is fun and challenging and fulfilling. I'd love knowing I have months at a time in one place, without the constant travel that comes with doing movies. In a sitcom you develop a very different circle of friends, people you build a rapport with and grow to trust, and it's so satisfying and secure. But if a sitcom doesn't work out, I'll find the next thing. There's always the next thing.

I'm not afraid of working hard or striving for things at this age. In fact, working hard is more pleasant these days, and far less pressured, because all the noise from the outside, all those *shoulds*, have been muted. And I don't follow anyone else's agenda—I work hard for the exact things I want . . . no more, and really, no less. Sure, there are still times I think about roads untaken, what could have been. But those musings are no longer accompanied by self-doubt. It's more like watching a *Sliding Doors* of my own life, and there are versions where maybe I got the part opposite Meryl Streep, but to even consider those versions means I have to consider the one where my star flamed out, or where I never discovered comedy. Sure, I can spend time wondering what could have been, but these days I find myself, far more often, wondering what might still be.

13

Minding My Own Business

STARTING SOMETHING NEW
WHEN THE WORLD SAYS YOU'RE TOO OLD

In my late forties, I did a Funny or Die video called "Starting Over." It was a pretend trailer for a pretend movie of the same name, in which I play high-powered businesswoman Miranda Huntington, who decides she needs a new lease on life. "Miranda Huntington was doing everything right," explains the dramatic voiceover. "But sometimes, doing it all right can leave you feeling all wrong."

Miranda Huntington leaves her job, and her husband, to start over as a candle shop owner, where she meets a sexy shirtless handyman, Roderigo, with whom she finds love . . . temporarily. Turns out, being a candle store owner isn't all it's cracked up to be. And so Miranda leaves that job, and that man, to open a vegan bakery. And then a video store. And then a kickboxing studio. And on and on, until Miranda Huntington ends up in prison, starting over once again.

The video is a hilarious spoof on the *Eat, Pray, Love* finding-one's-self trope, but it touches on something that is very real at this age. Not the desire to blow up a life or marriage or family, necessarily, but the urge to try something different. When I was first building the community that would lead me to launch Commence, a question I heard repeatedly from women was: "How do I start something new?" A new job, a new business, a new hobby, a new passion project. Women have hit the point where they're beginning to think about those dreams deferred, and they're wondering: If not now, when? And, at the same time, they're also wondering if they've already missed the boat. Is it too late?

For some of these women, the "something new" they dream of is to stop the merry-go-round altogether. They want to find low (or no) pressure ways to pay the rent and take it a bit easier. It's quite possible, and likely, that they've earned it. Any version of "starting over" counts.

I have not always wanted to be a business owner. This was not a lifelong dream that I finally mustered the courage to pursue. For me, Commence was the result of a confluence of factors. First of all, and most importantly, there was the frustration of being overlooked at the exact moment I was feeling in my prime, and the sense that there must be other women, across industries and lifestyles, feeling the same way. I wanted to connect with those women, and I knew I had acquired the platform over the years and the accompanying audience to foster that connection. I also knew that as an actress, professional opportunities were only going to get increasingly limited as I aged. Yes, there are the Helen Mirrens and Judi Denches and Vanessa Redgraves of the world, and they are amazing, and I remain their die-hard fan, but they're also the exceptions. Generally, the older you get, the less likely you are to get cast; there are simply fewer roles that call for your "type" (translation: your generation).

And it wasn't just acting roles. In 2022, I launched a podcast that a year and a half later I learned wasn't being renewed. (That was mostly a function of not meeting ad sales goals, which I get, but it's tough to get brands interested in the span of two seasons.) Then there was the day I was sitting on an airplane and opened Instagram only to see that True Botanicals, who hired me as a spokesperson in late 2021, had announced that the stunning, and ten years younger, Jessica Chastain was the new face of the brand. I had not even been told I was replaced and then eventually got the explanation that the brand evidently only hires their spokespeople for two years (would have been nice to know this ahead of time). Technically I wasn't being fired . . . my time had simply run its course. Well, well, well, didn't this seem to be the prevailing narrative?!

Though it may have been the natural culmination of my partnership with True Botanicals—but it was still a bit of an oh-shit moment. Jessica is absolutely lovely, and even more beautiful in person, if that is even possible, but my first thought was, *They moved on to a younger woman.* Across the board, as I get older, it feels like the opportunities coming my way are starting to dry up. Now, women over a certain age don't love to use the word "dry" to describe any part of ourselves or our lives, but what else was I supposed to think? If there was something I wanted to do, I'd need to have a clear plan and be more proactive.

This isn't just a Hollywood thing; a similar stalling, or limiting of opportunities, happens to women my age across industries. Research shows that pay growth for the average female worker peaks at age forty (for men, it's forty-nine).[1] A study in the *Harvard Business Review* notes that middle-aged women in the workplace are seen as "difficult to manage" and as having "too much family responsibility."[2] (No shit. Family responsibilities always fall to us. But that's what makes us such incredible multitaskers.) According to that study's authors: "One college leader described how some search committees chose not to hire women in their late forties because of 'too much family responsibility and impending menopause.' Other search committees declined to hire women in their fifties because they have 'menopause-related issues and could be challenging to manage.' . . . Yet the jobs were given to similarly aged men." IMPENDING MENOPAUSE!? This makes me crazy! It sounds like the End Times! How about impending penile dysfunction or the inevitable low ball sack? Citing impending menopause as prohibitive to being a qualified worker is like blaming women's emotions on being "on the rag." It's egregious and also . . . illegal? A combination of age and gender discrimination! Fuck these easy excuses for the patriarchy to count us as irrelevant or unnecessary. I should also point out that I could write an entirely separate book on how men, regardless of their age, are consistently challenging to manage. But I must refuse to lapse into bitterness or anger or victimhood. And this book is not about them (as so many things seem to be . . . oops, no lapsing, Brooke!). This is about us.

In other workplaces, the authors note, women of a certain age are seen as a liability because they're willing to stand up for themselves. The horror! Can you imagine? "As they do grow older and more mature in their careers, [women] lose some fear of speaking their mind. And certain men don't like that," Amy Diehl, one of the study's coauthors, told *HuffPost*.[3] Sound the distress alarm! "Men will allow women into the workplace . . . and will be supportive of women in the workplace to the extent that women are compliant, supportive of the men, and they don't push back." (Another finding of this study, which is less the case in Hollywood, was that basically, there is *no* good age to be a female employee. Women under forty in the traditional workplace are often dismissed as too young or too inexperienced and then—poof!— overnight they are too old.)

On top of all this, I am someone who craves creative fulfillment. I am completely positive I would not feel satisfied if I stopped working. It's a function of who I am at my core. Part of me envies those who don't have that same need. But for better or worse (and there is no better or worse—only choice or propensity) this is how I am wired.

Starting Commence was a way for me to harness my creativity as well as my experience and "iconography" (this word always makes my stomach hurt) and continue working in a way that wasn't hindered by my age but was actually served by it. I also love learning, and business was a frontier with which I had no experience. It was hard to resist the challenge of expanding my skill set and developing knowledge of a field that felt exciting and meaningful.

When people ask me for advice on starting something new in this phase of life, I don't have many words of wisdom beyond this: Just . . . start. They'll ask, "How did you find the courage?" and my answer is, "You can't think about it too much." Looking back, I waded into the business world rather blindly. I had no idea what I was getting into, or how hard it would be, but that naivete worked in my favor. I didn't know enough to know that I should be scared. The only thing I knew was that I couldn't do it alone, so my first step was to find someone who knew more than I did. I needed someone who understood the mission of the community I was envisioning and got me on a deeper level. When I found that person, I partnered with her. That's one real upside for starting a new endeavor in middle age: women are out there who've already done some version of what you want to do or who, on some level, are craving it. There are people you can learn from, people who can help you or work with you. And by this stage in life, you're savvy enough to surround yourself with experts and people who know what you do not. I had no problem asking for help from someone who knew the business world better than I did. There's a lot I still don't know at this stage, and I feel freed by acknowledging that.

My business partner, Karla De Bernardo, comes from corporate America. She worked at Kenneth Cole and Coach, and we were introduced by a mutual friend. We complement each other well—I came in passionate about the mission, with a strong platform and experience in connecting with women and being a voice for important issues; she similarly believed in the mission, but she also had the tactical business acumen. Her expertise is in business operations, and in what I have learned is called "concept to shelf." She knows how to take a product all the way through the manufacturing journey. For a while, it was just the two of us, figuring it all out together. I'd say "How do I build a website?" and then we'd call someone who I knew would have a recommendation. Then we had to incorporate, so we got a lawyer. We wanted to develop a brand identity, so we hired a creative director. That's how it went, step by step, one foot in front of the other. You ask one person you know and then talk to someone they recommend who connects you with someone else, and suddenly you've built a team, or at least the beginnings of one.

Starting a new business, versus a new hobby or new job, comes with the added burden of being expensive. When I had the idea for Commence, I had recently won a chunk of money in a lawsuit settlement. In early 2019, I was shopping with my daughters at Sephora when I came across a line of eyebrow pencils that were clearly named for different celebrities. There was the Grace K and the Naomi and the . . . Brooke S. *That's weird*, I thought. *I don't remember okaying that. Don't they need my permission before they can use my name to sell a product?* I'm known for my eyebrows—if someone is going to profit off them, shouldn't that person be me? I took a photo and sent it to my lawyer, explaining that I was no expert, but this seemed like it shouldn't be okay. "It is absolutely not okay," my lawyer immediately responded. We filed a lawsuit shortly thereafter and ended up settling later that year.

I used the money from that settlement to launch my business. It felt good to be able to fund my endeavor, at least at the beginning, with cash I made from sticking up for myself. I thought that by briefly funding myself, I got to avoid the hardest part. Plenty of people need to raise capital right away. And yet, I had so much to learn. While that lawsuit helped me over the hump of *one* hard part, I was completely naive about just how quickly any amount of money I invested would fly out the door. That settlement money only got us so far. Building a business is expensive! We needed a lot more cash than what I could offer, which meant we had to fundraise.

Asking for money is one of the hardest things I've had to do. I have experience pitching a television show, but that's a completely different beast—it's fast-paced and you do a bunch of pitches during a small window and that's it. It either sells or it doesn't. Raising capital for a company is more of a marathon, and it feels much more pressured. The conversations can be uncomfortable and people are skeptical, and I've had a lot of unpleasant exchanges with investors who are not shy about telling me all the things I should be doing differently (read: how they would do it). Also, I had no business experience! I'd get on Zoom calls with investors or advisors or potential team members who were throwing out terms like COGS and TAM and I'd be sitting there, googling definitions on my phone under the table. (COGS, I now know, is "cost of goods sold"; "TAM" is total addressable market. I'm learning!)

There were so many roadblocks as we continued to build this business, but whenever I'd voice my concerns, friends or acquaintances would say things like, "Of course you'll be able to raise the money—that's a no-brainer! You're Brooke Shields!" I always knew that wasn't the case. My name will get me the meeting—everyone wants to talk to a celebrity—but the idea that investors are going to fall all over themselves to give me money is misguided, and actually quite ignorant in my opinion. I knew that from the beginning. The "power of celebrity" needs much more strategy than one might think. I have seen it fail often. I, for one, have never led with celebrity because I understand its true lack of value. It's like expecting a TV show to be a huge success just because a famous actress is in it. She can bring in viewers to watch the first episode, but without talented writers to provide the actual material, a show can't succeed.

When it comes to business, celebrity can be a double-edged sword. People don't just go throwing their cash around, reasonably so, but there's also this assumption that celebrities who go into business are just in it because we need a fun hobby. A silly pet project. Or that it's really someone else's company and they just want to slap our face on it to help sell. Celebrities aren't always taken as seriously as other business owners (and, of course, female business owners are *already* taken less seriously in general—in 2022, companies led by all-women teams received about 2 percent of venture capital funding,[4] even though about 42 percent of all US businesses are owned by women).[5] Plus, venture capitalists want to invest money in companies where the CEO is going into the office every day and giving their attention to nothing but the business. That should not, in the long run, be me. I need to continue to keep what we jokingly refer to as "The Brooke Shields Machine" moving forward. I need to uphold the brand that has been building in one way or another since 1965. I am still going to perform and do speaking engagements and take spokesperson offers when they make sense. In a word, I still need to keep being BrookeShields—one word! We will undoubtedly hire a full-time CEO eventually, but not until I get us ready to grow even more successful.

I also am not best utilized only in an office every day. I love the idea of a beautiful desk and stunning view, like some role to be played, but I understand my value and the value of the experts around me. Still, it's hard not to resent it when potential investors ask, "How committed are you?" Obviously I'm committed. If I weren't, I wouldn't have spent hours upon hours on this, day in and day out, for the past five years. But instead of overtly bristling, I explain that I can understand their concern, but without the Brooke Shields they have come to know, the company would not exist. That said, it must never exist because of me alone. The power of Commence lies in the full team operating together and in all of us performing at our fullest capacities and with our collective and individual expertise.

Clearly, there has been a steep learning curve to my second act as a businesswoman. And, like I said, I'm glad I didn't anticipate how hard it would be, because I don't know if I'd have pursued it if I'd known more. There are moments when I absolutely wonder, *What was I thinking? The pressure is too much, why did I put myself through this?* And I can't say I wasn't warned. Every entrepreneur I spoke to when I was first starting out said the same thing: "Get ready. You are going to find yourself asking, time and again, why the hell did I do this? And yet something will power you through." I nervously laughed it off at the time, but I knew they were right. Sometimes I'll wake up in the night with an inkling of an idea for some aspect of the business, and that will keep me going. Or I'll be invited to speak at a conference on the topic of women and aging, and it'll serve as a reminder that people are hungry for this content. Or a new investor will sign on. Or someone will tell me the message resonates with them. Each of these moments is a little crumb, but they are enough sustenance to remind me that I'm in this for a reason. They're enough to keep me going.

Now, I want to be crystal clear. There are so many reasons why you might start a new endeavor. One is not more worthy than another. The fact that I believe there's a greater good to my work helps propel me, but that might be because I've spent a lifetime working in Hollywood. Obviously, the entertainment industry can have a positive impact, and I believe in the power of brilliant art, but there is a lot to it that is not necessarily geared toward helping people. Fame can be a ridiculous thing—it absolutely affords you privileges, but often those privileges only amount to a good seat at a restaurant or theater tickets. Nice perks, but they're not *important*, and I don't for a moment pretend that they are. Plus, it can all go away in an instant. As the saying goes, "you're only as good as your last job." So for me, working on something that's bigger than myself, something that gives voice to women's issues, has a lot of meaning.

That said, if you've spent your life working for others or serving them, it might be that the new endeavor you want to pursue is something that's purely for your own enjoyment. Starting an Etsy account to sell your art, maybe. Or joining a political campaign. Volunteering at the library. It might also be that you want to start a new job or new career path because you've found that at this age, there's extra pressure to create financial security for your future. Maybe you, like me, feel like your prospects in your current career are dwindling and you want or need to continue making a living. That's an important and valid reason! Maybe you're bored. Maybe you have more time because your kids went to college. It's all worthy. The idea that our age requires us to justify *why* we want to try something new is, in itself, a sign of a problem.

And so, whatever your reason, here you are. You want to start something new. And there are probably a million "buts" to scare you off. . . . *But* I've never done this before. *But* I'm too old. *But* I should have started a while ago, and now I've missed my chance. *But* I don't know enough. *But* I need a better reason than "I want to." (My butt, for one, scares me off from wearing bikinis, but I digress.) I'm not here to blindly root you on, or to say "you can do it!" with no context (even though, I feel confident, you can do it). But I absolutely believe that the only time it's too late to do something is when you're dead. If you really want to start a new job/hobby/company, you have to *really* want it, because at this age anything that is super hard or unpleasant isn't worth your time if there's not some valuable payout (monetary or otherwise). And, yes, ageism is still a very real factor in being able to start anew, and it may add some extra difficulty you don't deserve. But also, don't sell yourself short. You've lived a long time. You have experience. You can do hard things. You know more than you realize.

When we first started Commence, every time I had an idea or a notion of my next step, I would touch base with Karla for approval. Or maybe it was for validation or even permission. And every time, without fail, she would say, "You know this! You think because you didn't get a business degree you don't know what you're doing, but you have good instincts, and they haven't led you astray yet. Trust them." She had a point—truthfully, it had mostly been others' bad instincts that led me astray in my industry. When I actually followed my own, I was rarely sorry. It was exciting to hear Karla's words, because I have so much respect for her. And the business world, like most worlds, calls for a fake-it-till-you-make-it survival mentality. You can read books on how to create a startup, but every time I cracked one open, my eyes rolled into the back of my head. But still, you learn. You get thrown into rooms full of people and you're armed with only your PowerPoint presentation (to this day I'm not sure how to create one myself, but I can at least now understand one), and what other choice do you have but to make it work? Even that—the capacity to make it work—is something that comes with age and will serve you in whatever your next endeavor might be. You may not have experience in a specific field, but you know how to interact with other people. You know your strengths and your weaknesses. You've likely been the CEO of your household, planning schedules and mediating relationships, even if you didn't think to call it that.

When I think about my work at Commence—specifically about starting a company from nothing and with no startup experience, and now leading the team and asking for money—there is one thing I absolutely know for sure: I could not have done this when I was younger. First of all, I spent so many decades of my life following orders and doing what other people told me to do. It wasn't until I was in college that I realized I could have my own hypothesis rather than having to adopt the opinions of others, and it took even longer than that to find the courage to voice my opinions and stand by them. If you're sitting in a meeting with people who want you to prove the value of your company, you need to be able to state your case and back up your opinions.

Launching a business or asking for money also requires a thick skin. You won't always get the answers you want. It's logical to think that a career in entertainment would have gifted me with that armor from an early age—there's so much rejection in it, after all. But somehow I made it through Hollywood as sensitive as ever. Possibly even more so, because I've worked forever, and yet that doesn't make a difference where casting is concerned. My mother protected me from rejection and showered me with praise, so I didn't learn as a kid to hear a no and let it roll off my back. If I didn't get a part, I just thought I wasn't doing that particular job—maybe it was a scheduling conflict or not the right role. For a long time, it truly didn't occur to me that I had been passed over for someone else. This might have protected me from feeling bad in the short term, but it did not prepare me for the times when it was obvious I had gotten the Gong!

If I'd tried to start a business in my twenties, I wo
folded under the pressure. I needed to have childre
my mother, to go through the major milestones that
care less what other people thought of me. And to ful
and appreciate the fragility of life. I still get flustered ii
portant meetings, but now when I see myself getting un
can recover more quickly. The meetings get easier. You s
baby steps, and you realize, *Oh, I am able to voice my th*
do *know what I'm talking about. I do have opinions. We j*
more money. That's it. It's not personal! And if they don't
give it to us, we'll ask someone else. It really is that simple
may be the only simple thing about running a startup.

Across the board, entrepreneurs are better off when th
more decades under their belt. According to 2018 r
published in the *Harvard Business Review*, the average a
successful founder is forty-five.[6] Forget what you know
Mark Zuckerberg or Bill Gates or Steve Jobs—their stories
famous *because* they are unusual. "While young people ma
an edge creatively and technologically, their lack of indus
perience, as well as financial security, will [affect] their bu
success," wrote psychologist Sukanlaya Sawang in *The Con*
tion. "We gain knowledge and skills through both educatio
working experience."[7]

At this point, I've spent a lot of time sitting down with i
tors, walking them through the pitch, and explaining the
of our business. Over time, I began to recognize patterns. A
one is related to gender. As with any person raising money
business, we've gotten plenty of nos. Men and women have

us that, for whatever reason, they weren't going to give us money, at least not at the moment. Fine. That's par for the course. But the worst meetings, the ones that will always stick with me, have had nothing to do with the actual outcome, and everything to do with the way I was spoken to.

There was one particularly memorable meeting, a few months into our fundraising, where a man sitting across the table from us launched into a diatribe about everything Karla and I were doing wrong (according to him), down to the font size on our pitch deck. By that point, I'd learned a cardinal rule of pitching: You know within five minutes if they're going to invest. It's not unlike pitching a show to a network—pretty much immediately, the executives you're talking to are either riveted, smiling, and asking questions, or they're not so discreetly staring at their phones. An in-between apparently does not exist. By the time this guy (who had actually been fired from a very visible job in the beauty industry) began his rant, I'd been through the song and dance enough times to know how feedback was usually delivered. This was not it. I'd had enough of the mansplaining and the condescension, but I maintained composure and a level of respect that made me proud. Still, I had to respond. "You know, the crazy thing is," I began, "I'm asking you for money, I'm not asking you for your opinion."

He got a little flustered and started backpedaling. "Well . . . I just . . . I've had a lot of experience so I'm just giving you my advice."

"I'm just giving you a hard time," I said with a laugh. "We know your time is valuable and don't wish to waste any of it." I know how to play this game. Being that straightforward isn't the way to win with someone like this. As author and organizational psychologist Adam Grant wrote in a *New York Times* editorial: "Disclaimers (I might be wrong, but . . .), hedges (maybe, sort

of), and tag questions (don't you think?) can be a strategic advantage."[8] As I often find myself telling the audience at various professional women's events, we can try to be the loudest voice in the room, but I find there are better ways to outsmart the guys. If I come at a potential investor too hot, he immediately gets ready for a pissing contest. When you're dealing with so-called alpha males, they don't really want to hear your good counterpoints *or* your anger. But if I take a more nuanced approach, speaking the way they expect or letting them start with a win, I think of it as the smarter way to maneuver.

It sounds like playing games, perhaps, but I think of it more as being strategic. It may sound antifeminist, but I don't have any problems playing a man's game because I know I'm going to play it better, precisely because I have no ego about *how* I come out on top. In his op-ed, Grant suggests that the goal should be not to change our language but to alter what we consider "antifeminist." He writes: "The solution is to normalize 'weak language' as a strong way to express concern and humility. If we do that, we won't have to keep encouraging women to communicate more forcefully. Instead, we'll finally be able to recognize the difference between assertiveness and aggressiveness." It's like chess—I may appear weak or subservient in the moment, but it's all a tactic. Beating men at their own game is, I believe, one of the most feminist things you can do.

The truth is, when I told this investor that I didn't want his opinion, I meant it. If he didn't like what we presented, or how we answered his questions, he had every right to pass. He didn't, on the other hand, have every right to talk to me like I was an idiot. Obviously, if he had wanted to invest but also had well-earned advice to share, we would have listened. That's how we have gotten this far. We value our investors and their expertise, and trust that they're in the trenches with us. And certainly not every meeting with a male investor has ended this way, but it wasn't an isolated incident either (though I never used that "I want your money, not your opinion" line again—it did feel a bit inappropriate. But I had read the room, and because I recovered well, no bridges were burned). Condescension has been a common theme, but it is something that no longer intimidates me. Also, it's important to note that not all money is the right money. Just because you're offered an investor's cash doesn't mean that person is a good fit. After leaving many a meeting, Karla and I have looked at each other and said: "Nope, that is not a person we want to be in business with." We always seem to be on the same page with those assessments.

I've also had issues with potential investors who assume their involvement will translate to unlimited access to me at all times. Having 24/7 access to a CEO is never guaranteed to any investor. And no one would demand that of a man in my position. It just wouldn't seem reasonable. Yes, if someone supports your business they should feel free to reach out when they have a concern, but the idea that any businessperson will drop everything the second an investor calls is unreasonable. Still, had this happened a couple of decades ago, I would have basically said, "Sure, what do you need from me? What can I give you and what can you take?"

Even when they are productive, I've found that for me, business meetings with men—not always, but often—take about fifteen minutes to truly get underway. Sometimes I'll say to Karla, "Watch for it, they'll spend the first fifteen minutes just processing me," and it might seem weird, but they have to get the Brooke Shields piece out of their system. I bluff through it with small talk, because by fifteen minutes in, the judgment and scrutiny is over and we can finally have a real conversation.

Karla and I sat down with two female investors the other day. They listened carefully to our pitch and asked great questions when they wanted to understand more about the community or the financials. They waited for us to inquire before they offered their opinions, and the feedback they shared was constructive and delivered respectfully. They took a completely different approach than did so many of the men we've pitched, and I found it remarkable, because they didn't make it about them, even though they were in the exact demo and life experience we are targeting as a business. It actually *was* about them! They were uniquely qualified to tell us what, if anything, we were doing wrong, and yet they had no interest in doing so. Certainly we've met with other women who've been tough and discerning, but they too have treated us as equals. With the female investors we consistently felt respected, and we've always learned from our discussions. They've set a professional tone and always provided helpful notes.

When you start something new at any age, there's no guarantee it will work out. It could fail entirely, or morph into something different from what you originally intended. When I first started Commence, I thought I wanted to focus only on community. Product wasn't at the top of the list, but one of the most-asked questions I got from day one was about my hair. This has always been my "thing"—my long locks, my thick eyebrows. But in middle age, hair quality changes a lot. It thins, it grays, it gets drier. Scalp health deteriorates. Since it kept coming up, Karla and I did the research and learned that there was a white space in the market when it came to aging hair. There was hair dye, or shampoo that was "color-safe," but no one was addressing women over forty and the needs of their scalp health and hair in particular. We decided that shifting into beauty, and hair care specifically, made sense for our business. It was a shift that emerged directly from our community's concerns—it served a need but was also a natural fit based on my history. We maintained our connection with our community but also started focusing on specific needs women have regarding their scalp and hair. We hired an expert product formulator, developed a line that served the hair needs of women over forty, and eventually relaunched with a shift in focus.

I won't pretend I'm immune to the fear of failure, but I've learned by now how to sit in that fear and tolerate it, rather than let it drive me away from something I want. And if a new endeavor does go up in smoke . . . well, we've all lived through worse.

I did a pilot a couple of years ago. In it, I played a big-time intimidating CEO. While we were filming, I struggled a bit with being demonstrative and scary because it was so not in my nature. I decided that I actually did not want to play the part. I think about that role from time to time these days, because if I had the experience I have now, of being a CEO, I think I would have understood her better and played the part stronger. I don't rule Commence with an iron fist, but I have a clearer understanding of what it takes to run a company. Today I call myself a businesswoman without feeling like I'm lying. I am no longer plagued by impostor syndrome. I don't know how it will all work out—I would love for the company to outlast me and become a household name—but I don't kid myself about what a lofty goal that is. Still, our products are on sale today. We did that. Sometimes I still don't know how, but we did it. All because I thought, *Why not*, when everyone else was asking, *Why now*.

14

The Good Part

ON MOVING FORWARD

received an unexpected invitation recently. I was asked to join
Meghan Markle and Katie Couric, as well as sociologist Nancy
Wang Yuen, in a discussion moderated by journalist Errin
Haines at a South by Southwest (SXSW) keynote panel. The
conversation, which took place on International Women's Day,
was titled "Breaking Barriers, Shaping Narratives: How Women
Lead on and off the Screen." It was a flattering invitation, and my
younger self might have responded in one of a few ways. I might
have said yes out of obligation—when Katie Couric asks you to
do something, when the Duchess of Sussex comes calling, you say
yes—and then panicked out of fear that I didn't belong. I might
have made myself smaller and politely declined because I felt
like I didn't have enough to offer. But when the ask came in, my
first thought was, *Wow, I'm onto something. What I stand for and
what I'm putting out there—this message about womanhood and
aging—it's getting traction. We have something that people crave.*

I accepted the invitation, not because I had to, or because I
thought I could leverage it in some way that would benefit me
personally, but because I had something to say regarding breaking barriers and shaping narratives. I accepted because I was invited, so obviously somebody thought I belonged there. And I

accepted because I wanted to be there—I thought it would be an interesting discussion. I thought it would be a great platform for engaging in this conversation around women and aging, and figured I might even learn a few things in the process.

When I do panels like this, I'm often asked for my best advice— for aging gracefully, for handling doubts, for finding balance, for dealing with those who don't want you to change. And you'd think that after nearly six decades I'd have plenty of wisdom to impart, and lessons to share. But I'm no fool. If I've learned anything as I've aged it's that telling people how to live their lives doesn't work. It never has the intended effect. Plus, who am I to claim to be an expert on anything for anybody but myself? My goal has never been to tell people to do what I do, or to look like me, or to do as I say. In my opinion, too many famous people believe they are experts on something just because they're famous.

More often than not, when a friend comes to me for advice, what they're really asking for is validation that their opinion is best, or confirmation that whatever they've already done was the right thing to do. They're looking for forgiveness, or a pat on the back. In a moderated discussion in any public forum, when I'm asked for advice, I usually deflect and instead simply share what I did in a similar situation, why it worked, or what I wish I'd done differently. People can take from my personal experiences what they want. Or I answer by asking questions of whoever it is that needs help so that they can hear their own responses and reflect and figure out what they want for themselves. It sounds like an annoying therapist's response, but I have come to believe that in order to grow we need to continue to get in touch with our honest selves. It's like telling an alcoholic they need to stop drinking for you. It never works. They need to want to do it for themselves. The minute you say to someone "you know what you should do . . ." you're assigning them a task, and if they fail at said task, it usually just makes the current problem even worse. But saying "well, what does your gut tell you?" can be much more productive—it can help them learn for themselves and maybe not make the same mistake again. Even with my kids I try not to advise on what they *should* do in a tough situation so much as say, "I'm so sorry you're feeling this way, the one thing I can promise you is that it won't always hurt this much. It won't always feel like this." Then we discuss what might be going on with the person who hurt them or why something difficult happened. This kind of conversation is definitely more work and a bit more exhausting, and it's probably so much easier to just judge and bark orders, but it doesn't help our kids learn and grow and deal with life. (People say "oh, to be young again," but I would never go back to my early twenties. That pain is real.)

It's funny how the older we get, the more we understand how much we don't know. I'm not delusional enough to think I have life figured out. The only time I've dispensed advice in a book is when I was in college, when I was young enough to know nothing but think I knew everything. That book, *On Your Own*, offered life lessons about the best way to apply mascara and other similarly weighty matters. Even the term "life lessons" being applied to a barely eighteen-year-old is a laugh. (In my defense, I was asked to write a book about the transition to adulthood, and after turning in my first chapter, the publisher told me I was going too deep, and it would be best if I stuck to topics like how best to wear leg warmers or choose what to eat at a deli salad bar.) Still, college was a period where I began to think that maybe people in my life *could* use my advice. I took a bunch of psych classes, and like every college student who has taken Psych 101, I fancied myself a therapist. I'd be talking with a friend who'd mention a problem she was having, and because I wanted to make everything better for her, I would share my knowledge and dispense my opinion on what she should do next. Well, it turned out she hadn't asked for my advice! And she most likely didn't want it. She just wanted a friend to listen. I find this happens often in my marriage, but the other way around. I'll feel the need to vent to my husband, and he'll feel the need to fix it all. But what I really want is for someone to hear me and support me. And to hear myself out loud, so that I can discover what I need to do in that situation.

The older I get, the less equipped I feel to tell others how to live. I can share my personal stories, but there are endless ways to be a woman of a certain age in America. I know only one of them. Some of what I've experienced is rather commonplace; other parts of my life have been quite extraordinary. But there are aspects of aging in this country that I believe connect all of us middle-aged women. Society's pervasive disregard of our existence is a big one. Nothing brings a group together like being underestimated. But I think we are also connected by our sense of power, and our determination to dismantle this outdated notion of what it means to be a mature woman. Every time I sit down at a conference or a panel or a gathering where there's an audience full of women in this phase of life, the concept of power comes up repeatedly. It's embodied by the intelligence and the multitasking ability and the confidence that emerge in this moment. It's embodied by our shared excitement and determination and curiosity and fearlessness and fuck-it-why-not attitude. It's embodied, if nothing else, by the growing number of women in the seats.

I once had the honor of listening to Nelson Mandela speak during a visit to Africa. Someone in the audience asked him how he managed to stay positive during all those years he was imprisoned, and he told us the story of an afternoon when he heard two guards outside his cell arguing about apartheid. The mere fact that there was an argument meant that something was brewing. That stuck with me. I'm not comparing myself to Nelson Mandela by any means—let's all be clear on that, okay?—but I think about that story, and that seed of hope, so often these days. Because the ways we regard aging in this country are not going to change overnight. Our attitudes toward women who can no longer bear children won't suddenly do a 180. But the fact that people are talking about these issues, that women are gathering, that maybe there are small arguments happening in households across the country, or women sticking up for themselves—it's a sign. Something is brewing.

Every time I've decided to discuss "women's issues" publicly—postpartum depression, the sexualization of young girls, aging, the list goes on—what I've been most struck by is the community that forms around the conversation. The sense of unity that comes from talking about our experiences. Once you verbalize your struggle, you give people who are dealing with something similar a context to coexist. It is so important to be able to acknowledge the validity of your experience, and one way to do that is by seeing yourself in someone else's story. It makes you feel less alone on your journey. I'm honored to offer that support to people in some small way. But I don't presume to know anyone's life better than they do.

Just as I'm reluctant to offer advice, I'll admit I'm very selective about receiving it. There are a few people whose opinions I value, and I share with them when I'm struggling with a decision or dealing with a tough moment with my kids or in my marriage or in my career. I admire the way they walk through life, so understanding how they might handle a situation can be enlightening. But the most empowering thing about this age, truly, is that I've lived long enough to trust myself. I know what I know, and I know a lot. I know the values I want to live by and the way I want to behave. I know how it feels when I shrink myself to accommodate someone else. When I do something because I figure I *should* rather than because it will benefit me in some way. If I really stop and listen to myself, I usually know how I want to move forward in any given moment, what will sit right with me and what will not.

I was recently part of a team of actors and producers who were pitching a sitcom to a bunch of different networks. We practiced the pitch ahead of time, and I was told, essentially, to be seen and not heard. The producer would give the pitch, I would mostly just smile, and then I would answer questions when they came up. Well, the pitch sucked. I hate to say that, because it's a project I was excited about, but anyone sitting in those Zoom meetings could tell they weren't going well. I kept texting the producer on the side, asking *Please, can I chime in?* Every time, the answer was the same: let them ask questions and then you can say more. Well, no one was asking questions, so I never got a chance to say much of anything, and the meetings came and went with no deal in place. And rather than ever saying "you were right" or "maybe we should have given you a chance," the response I got was . . . "bummer." Oh boy was I seeing red!

Now, I'm not saying that I could have swooped in and saved the meeting or sold the sitcom on the strength of my charisma or powers of persuasion. It's entirely possible, maybe even likely, that I would have jumped in and said my piece and the outcome of the pitch would have been the same. But who knows? I would have at least gotten a chance to bat (notice the strong use of a sports analogy! It's baseball, right?). I should not have let someone tell me when I could and could not speak, but I fell into an old habit of obedience, and afterward all I could think was,

Brooke, you know better. Never again will I be told to stay quiet or be smaller.

I may be older and wiser, but change is hard, and this was an important reminder of how I want to live my life at this stage. Every step of the way, I could see the problems clear as day, and when I spoke up, I was told to "let it play out." That kind of passivity doesn't work for me anymore. I believe in my instincts. I believe in my gut. I believe in my own knowledge and experience. Next time, I promised myself, I will speak. That doesn't mean I'm going to yell over people or cut others off or make something The Brooke Show when I'm working with a team. But I can make my voice heard. Even if it doesn't work out, I would rather speak up than let myself get cut off at the knees by somebody who assumes he knows better.

And so, when I arrived in Austin, Texas, for SXSW, I did better. During our panel, I sat on the stage alongside Meghan and Katie, and at one point, Meghan told the story of how, when she was eleven, she wrote to Procter & Gamble to complain about an ad for their Ivory Clear dishwashing soap. "The gloves are coming off—women are fighting greasy pots and pans with Ivory Clear," the ad said. Meghan wrote to the company to ask them to change "women" to "people," and they did. She mentioned multiple times that she was only eleven when this happened, so I couldn't resist jumping in. I raised my hand and said, "Excuse me, but I have to just mention something, to just show you how Meghan and I differ. . . . When I was eleven, I was playing a prostitute!" Then I added, "I wish I had known you when I was eleven!" The whole place erupted into laughter.

It was just a funny aside. The panel was so serious, and we could have so quickly devolved into doom and gloom and politics and hardship and pity, with the main takeaway being all the ways we've been mistreated as women. And those are all important points, but I also don't want to lose sight of the excitement and opportunity we have as older women. About the joy! I think it's always quite disarming when a serious message can be coupled with some levity. I know there are probably people who thought I should have sat back and kept my mouth shut, but this was not the time nor the place to temper my instincts. This was the exact environment to switch up the way we are perceived as women of a certain age. We are in this phase together. I thought, *Why not let loose a bit and see the reaction? I know how to address this crowd, be respectful to the other panelists, be myself, and still be effective.* And it worked! We lightened the mood, brought the crowd together, and created a relaxed nonjudgmental environment, all the while fighting for progress.

Recently, I went to see a podiatrist, because I was in a lot of pain when I walked. (As mentioned, I've long had problems with my feet. One time a girlfriend looked at my bare feet, aghast, and said, "What happened? God got to your feet and just said, 'Fuck it, I'm tired'?" In fact, in some of the promotional images for my recent Netflix movie, *Mother of the Bride*, I'm standing barefoot. It's set on a beach in Thailand, after all. I took one look at the photos and immediately called the director. "Those aren't my toes," I said. He inhaled audibly over the phone. "Yeah," he said. "We had to CGI your toes.") I've had so many surgeries on them already, and I'm not getting any younger. So I asked her, is the surgery worth doing? Or is this just an occupational hazard of getting older?

"Oh God no," she said. "It's not like you're ninety! You have years of moving still ahead. You need to be able to walk pain free!"

It was so refreshing, and a good reminder that despite what society would have us believe, women of a certain age are not washed up or past our prime or at the end. We have plenty of life ahead of us. There is no reason to accept a lesser version of that life, even if conventional wisdom has taught us that we should simply take what we can get, or be grateful just to be here.

If I had to point to a piece of great advice I've gotten recently, that would be it: keep moving. Walk without pain or shame. Do not accept less for your life.

When we were designing the packaging for our Commence products, we worked with a design team called Established. There was a woman working the elevator and manning the front desk in the lobby of the building where we met to create our designs, and from the first moment I laid eyes on her I noticed how stunning she was. She had an incredible energy. She was chic, and she sparkled when she smiled. At work, she met every visitor to the building with a nod and a kind word and a consistent knowledge of what floor they were visiting. She just brightened the day. Once we got to talking, I learned she was seventy-five and from Trinidad. She'd been a competitive sprinter her whole life. When it came time to shoot our campaign, we decided to invite her to participate. Thankfully she said yes, and unsurprisingly, she was a natural in front of the camera. "I have to introduce her to my agent," one of our other models said. Now this woman is seventy-six and has the potential for an entirely new career path—every time I see her she's glowing with possibility. That is what Commence is all about, and what I hope this stage is about for all women. Not getting discovered for a second act as a model, necessarily, but being open to new experiences. Knowing that new opportunities are out there. Understanding that there is power in this stage, and having the conviction to step into it.

've been thinking a lot about the "what's next" of it all. Because like my doctor said, it's not like I'm ninety (and even ninety today is not what it used to be). I've still got a lot of growing and learning and changing to do. The beauty of it is that I don't have to answer to anyone but myself. Yes, there are people who love me and root for me and even a few who rely on me, but I trust myself more to help make the best decisions for all of us.

Here's another invitation I got recently: to appear alongside Cynthia Erivo and Susan Boyle in three performances and a recording of Sondheim's *A Little Night Music* with a sixty-piece orchestra. I was incredibly flattered and accepted the invitation immediately. These are the kinds of vocal powerhouses I was punishing myself to measure up to in those early days of rehearsals at The Carlyle. To be considered in their company was no small thing.

But then I took my pulse on the offer. How was I feeling about this opportunity? Panicked? Definitely. Terrified? Sure. Excited? Actually . . . no. The only emotions I could access were negative—stress, nerves, fear. I knew it would be hard, and that I probably wouldn't kill in it, and that I'd be so nervous that I'd only feel relief when it was over. The performance itself would probably be wonderful—I couldn't wait to see it myself—but I could tell that my anxiety around it would completely overshadow any joy I might get from being a part of it and no doubt hurt my own ability to be at my best. It would take time and energy from my life to fully prepare and mostly deliver stress in return. I would also probably continue to play the old tapes in my head, shouting that I would never be as strong a singer as anybody else on the stage. Which is true, and okay. I had talents that meant I would deserve to be there. And I knew I could work my way up to being stronger vocally than I had ever been. But I didn't think it was an environment that was really suited to what I do best. It wasn't a musical theater production where I could sing and dance and be comedic. It was a bona fide Sondheim concert. I am not a concert performer, nor have I ever tried to be. I knew I'd beat myself up and get insecure and undo so much of the confidence I have worked for in my life and career. Ultimately, I had to ask myself only one question: Do I want to do this? The answer was, quite obviously, no. I wanted to have done it, which is never a good enough reason to do a project.

I pulled out of the performance. I did so professionally, and with more than enough time for them to find a replacement before rehearsals began, but the sheer relief I felt after withdrawing from the project told me all I needed to know. If I'd stuck with it, I would have made it through. Maybe I would have even surprised myself—or surprised audiences and critics alike!—but so what? I kept thinking about the job, with terror and trepidation, and finally I got there. *Why do I need to put myself through this? What am I trying to prove?* And so I said thanks but no thanks. I will enjoy watching the show much more from the audience, so that's what I plan to do.

Do I want to do this? If I had to boil down the joy and freedom of aging to one question, that would be it. The fact that I'm finally at a place where I can ask myself if I want something, answer honestly, and act accordingly—that's the joy of this time. And I'm not talking just about work. I'm lucky to have the ability to say no to professional offers, but this mindset applies to everything else, too—who you allow into your life, or how you pass your very valuable downtime. I can now make decisions that make sense for me, professionally *and* personally. I can decide that I only want to pursue endeavors that I'm excited about, or that have real purpose. It could be that I've always wanted to visit a certain city, so sure, I'll take on a speaking engagement there. Or that I don't particularly enjoy that person so, no, I'll pass on the dinner with them. I can decide to do something I'm scared of, if I actually want to, despite the insecurities that are always lurking. Whenever we put Tuzi outside to go pee, she does her business and ends up standing at the door, with her paws up and her nose against the window, just waiting to be let back in. "You're like my insecurities!" I tell her. "Always at the ready!" They're there, but I don't want to waste my time giving them any attention. Unlike my adorable pup, who I will always let in, and shower with love.

There's a moment in *Love Letters* where John Slattery's character, Andrew Makepeace Ladd III, is talking about rowing, and how there seems to be no rhyme or reason to who succeeds and who doesn't. "I went to Mr. Clark who is the head of rowing and I said, 'Look, Mr. Clark. There's something wrong about this system. People are constantly moving up and down and no one knows why. It doesn't seem to have anything to do with whether or not you're good or bad, strong or weak, coordinated or uncoordinated. It all seems random, sir.' And Mr. Clark said, 'That's life, Andy.' And walked away." Andy goes on to contend that life doesn't have to be that way. There could be rules, where the good guys move up and the bad ones move down, and everyone understands what's happening. When I did the play this last time, Andy's rowing rant really spoke to me. His is an optimistic way of looking at the world. When you're young—which Andy is when he delivers these lines—it's comforting to assume the world could be so reasonable and fair. And yet, as a woman in her fifties, I know better. Because just as I was feeling stronger and more confident, surer that what I had to offer the world was richer than what I've offered in the past, my value started to dissipate. At the exact moment when I was doing really well, I got sent down two crews.

How we deal with the knowledge that life follows no logical system, that we are being sent down two crews despite how hard we've worked, is how we exert our power. Personally, I've chosen to respond by rejecting the notion that I should back into the bushes like Homer Simpson in that ubiquitous meme. The more I'm expected to be invisible, to make no demands, or to fade away so that I can be frozen in time as a specific (read: younger) version of Brooke Shields, the more fully I intend to stand tall and take up space as the woman I am now.

I had lunch the other day with Lisa, my best friend from high school, and Karla, my business partner. We were talking about all the obstacles that can make this time of life tricky. "You forget that you matter," Lisa said. This, from a woman who has four children. Who supports another family member. Who runs a huge company. She matters. But we live in a culture that doesn't always remind you, one that's perfectly happy to let you forget.

Fuck that. There's probably a more eloquent way to say that, but another thing age has taught me is not to use five words when two will do. We matter. Our needs matter and our desires matter and I can only care so much if the men out there or the twenty-somethings or the marketers ever fully wake up to that fact. Of course that would be ideal, but I can't sit around and wait for the outside world to start to make changes that I can make for myself. I have to take the reins.

What I care about, above all else, is that we all remember that we matter. That we aren't tricked into believing the stories meant to diminish us. I care that we keep growing. Maturing with ownership and agency and knowing the full extent of our value and power is liberating. But I hope we can also have fun along the way. Because aging isn't just "better than the alternative," as the saying goes. It's better than what came before. I won't pretend my knees don't ache on occasion, or that I don't have a Rolodex full of doctors and specialists. (Even a Rolodex reference is from a bygone era, but I still like it.) But I don't have the worries I used to. I've prioritized joy, which I hardly used to care about, because I found it so fleeting. I took everything so seriously back then. My profession. My craft. My reputation. My existence. And yet I don't have advice for my younger self, because I needed to go through all that to get to this place of freedom and fun and empowerment and strength. I've paid plenty of dues, as we all have, and there will likely be more. What matters is that now I'm here. And I plan to enjoy myself.

ACKNOWLEDGMENTS

I want to thank Bob Miller for always believing in me and the stories I needed to share. I will follow you wherever you go. I also want to thank Rachel Bertsche for understanding my voice often before I did, and Julie Will for her unbiased and insightful editing. Thank you to the literary department at UTA—Albert Lee, Pilar Queen, Nancy Gates—for saying, "Hey, what are your thoughts about writing a book about this era of your life?"

There are so many other individuals who have worked on and committed to this book, many of whom I have never even met. To the entire team at Flatiron Books, including Marlena Bittner, Cat Kenney, Nancy Trypuc, Maris Tasaka, Guy Oldfield, Deborah Feingold, Keith Hayes, Emily Walters, and Sydney Jeon; thank you for paying attention to the details and for actually caring.

To Jill Fritzo, thanks for masterminding every press tour and making me feel like I'm never alone . . . and, of course, for the snacks.

To Karla De Bernardo, aka "Joey," thank you for jumping into this difficult journey with me. You make me stronger and more confident every day. I'm proud of us. We are just COMMENCING.

To Caitlin Simpson, my personal assistant and actual "boss," for being in on the joke and for making every "less-than-ideal" situation manageable . . . and for your radiant smile.

To my soul girlfriends (you know who you are) for being exactly where we are and saying "fuck it, let's keep going" . . . and laughing at the craziness of it all. And to Lyda, who was in the rooms when my girls were born and who has been mentioned in every one of my books—for fifty-nine years (and nine months!) you have been a loyal friend, and I am forever grateful.

To my patient husband, Chris, who inherited a lot when we fell in love: You are the pain in the ass I would not want to live without. Thank you for your humor and for constantly encouraging me to be my best self. See, I too am figuring it out! Thank goodness for you and the long haul.

To my incredible girls, Rowan and Grier: You have grown into strong, funny, independent young women. I am in awe and so proud of who you are. I love you so much it "HORTS!" Thank you for loving me back.

NOTES

INTRODUCTION

1. Kirsten Weir, "Ageism Is One of the Last Socially Acceptable Prejudices. Psychologists Are Working to Change That," *Monitor on Psychology* 54, no. 2 (March 1, 2023). https://www.apa.org/monitor/2023/03/cover-new-concept-of-aging.
2. Katie Keating, "What Women over 40 Are Worth to Your Marketing Mix," LinkedIn, August 26, 2021. https://www.linkedin.com/pulse/what-women-over-40-worth-your-marketing-mix-katie-keating/
3. Girl Power Marketing, "Statistics on the Purchasing Power of Women." https://girlpowermarketing.com/statistics-purchasing-power-women/.
4. Katie Keating, "1 in 4 Americans Is a Woman over 40. So Why Do So Many Feel Ignored?" *Fast Company*, July 1, 2021. https://www.fastcompany.com/90649731/1-in-4-americans-is-a-woman-over-40-so-why-do-so-many-feel-ignored.
5. Sara Karlovitch, "Advertising Returns to Depicting Women More Frequently in Domestic Roles, Study Finds," *Marketing Dive*, March 10, 2023. https://www.marketingdive.com/news/gender-diversity-advertising-spend/644657/.
6. Zoe Caplan, "U.S. Older Population Grew from 2010 to 2020 at Fastest Rate Since 1880 to 1890," U.S. Census Bureau, May 25, 2023. https://www.census.gov/library/stories/2023/05/2020-census-united-states-older-population-grew.html.
7. Katie Keating, "Brands Continue to Overlook Women over 40 as a Group Worth Marketing To," *Adweek*, March 6, 2019. https://www.adweek.com/agencies/brands-continue-to-overlook-women-over-40-as-a-group-worth-marketing-to/.

1: PREVIOUSLY OWNED BY BROOKE SHIELDS

1. "Fail, Frumpy and Forgotten: A Report on the Movie Roles of Women of Age." Retrieved from https://geenadavisinstitute.org/wp-content/uploads/2024/01/frail-frumpy-and-forgotten-report.pdf.
2. Elizabeth Arias, Kenneth D. Kochanek, Jiaquan Xu, and Betzaida Tejada-Vera, "Provisional Life Expectancy Estimates for 2022," Centers for Disease Control and Prevention, Vital Statistics Rapid Release No. 31 (November 2023). https://www.cdc.gov/nchs/data/vsrr/vsrr031.pdf.
3. Martha M. Lauzen, "Boxed In: Women on Screen and Behind the Scenes on Broadcast and Streaming Television in 2021-22," San Diego State Center

for the Study of Women in Television and Film, https://womenintvfilm.sdsu
.edu/wp-content/uploads/2022/10/2021-22-Boxed-In-Report.pdf.

4. Patricia Lippe Davis, "Why Marketers Should Be Scared of Ignoring 50-Plus
   Women," *Campaign Live*, October 31, 2018. https://www.campaignlive.com
   /article/why-marketers-scared-ignoring-50-plus-women/1497689.

5. Lisa Anderson, "It's Official: Many Women Become Invisible After 49,"
   Reuters, April 13, 2015. https://www.reuters.com/article/idUSKBN0N41RG/.

6. Susan Dominus, "Women Have Been Misled About Menopause," *New York
   Times*, February 1, 2023. https://www.nytimes.com/2023/02/01/magazine
   /menopause-hot-flashes-hormone-therapy.html.

7. Ali Rogin and Claire Mufson, "Menopause Is Ubiquitous, So Why Is It
   Often Stigmatized and Ignored?" *PBS NewsHour*, April 30, 2023. https://
   www.pbs.org/newshour/show/menopause-is-ubiquitous-so-why-is-it-often
   -stigmatized-and-ignored.

8. Melissa Lee Phillips, "The Mind at Midlife," *Monitor on Psychology* 42, no.
   4 (April 2011). https://www.apa.org/monitor/2011/04/mind-midlife.

9. Tara Parker-Pope, "The Midlife Crisis Goes Global," *New York Times*,
   January 30, 2008. https://archive.nytimes.com/well.blogs.nytimes.com/2008
   /01/30/the-midlife-crisis-goes-global.

2: NOT BACKING DOWN, NOT BACKING OUT

1. "Symptoms of Depression Among Women," Centers for Disease Control
   and Prevention, https://www.cdc.gov/reproductive-health/depression
   /index.html.

2. *Ypulse*, "The Confidence Code for Girls: The Confidence Collapse and
   Why It Matters for the Next Gen," https://static1.squarespace.com
   /static/588b93f6bf629a6bec7a3bd2/t/5ac39193562fa73cd8a07a89
   /1522766258986/The+Confidence+Code+for+Girls+x+Ypulse.pdf.

3. "Survey Reveals That American Women Are Aging Beautifully; Good Hair
   Days Boost Confidence," *PR Newswire*, October 17, 2023. https://www
   .prnewswire.com/news-releases/survey-reveals-that-american-women-are
   -aging-beautifully-good-hair-days-boost-confidence-301958303.html.

4. Anya Meyerowitz, "Two-Thirds of Women Are Significantly More Self-
   Confident When They Reach This Age," *Red*, March 8, 2019. https://www
   .redonline.co.uk/red-women/news-in-brief/a26762673/self-confidence-age/.

5. Joe Folkman, "How Women in Leadership Demonstrate and Cultivate
   Confidence," *Zenger Folkman*, June 13, 2023. https://zengerfolkman.com
   /articles/how-women-in-leadership-demonstrate-and-cultivate-confidence/.

6. Jack Zenger and Joe Folkman, "How Age and Gender Affect Self-
   Improvement," *Harvard Business Review*, January 5, 2016. https://hbr.org
   /2016/01/how-age-and-gender-affect-self-improvement.

7. Jennifer A. Chatman, Daron Sharps, Sonya Mishra, Laura J. Kray, and
   Michael S. North, "Agentic but Not Warm: Age-Gender Interactions and
   the Consequences of Stereotype Incongruity Perceptions for Middle-Aged
   Professional Women," *Organizational Behavior and Human Decision Processes* 173 (November 2022). https://www.sciencedirect.com/science/article
   /pii/S0749597822000796.

3: CHARACTER STUDY

1. Paul Nelson, "Study: Women Don't Give Themselves Enough Credit at Work," KSL.com, August 13, 2009. https://www.ksl.com/article/7517173/study-women-dont-give-themselves-enough-credit-at-work.

2. Christina Pazzanese, "Women Less Inclined to Self-Promote Than Men, Even for a Job," *Harvard Gazette*, February 7, 2020. https://news.harvard.edu/gazette/story/2020/02/men-better-than-women-at-self-promotion-on-job-leading-to-inequities/.

3. Ashley Batts Allen and Mark R. Leary, "Self-Compassionate Responses to Aging," *The Gerontologist* 54, no. 2 (April 2014): 190–200. https://www.ncbi.nlm.nih.gov/pmc/articles/PMC3954413/.

4. Social Security Administration. Actuarial Life Table. https://www.ssa.gov/oact/STATS/table4c6.html.

5. Josh Wright, "What Is the Power of Regret? A Conversation with Daniel Pink," *Behavioral Scientist*, December 13, 2022. https://behavioralscientist.org/what-is-the-power-of-regret-a-conversation-with-daniel-pink/.

4: BRADLEY COOPER, GUARDIAN ANGEL

1. Awais Aftab et al., "Meaning in Life and Its Relationship with Physical, Mental, and Cognitive Functioning," *Journal of Clinical Psychiatry* 81, no. 1 (December 2019). https://www.psychiatrist.com/jcp/meaning-in-life-and-physical-mental-and-cognitive-functioning/.

5: NO LONGER THE PUNCHING BAG

1. Teresa Thomas et al., "A Conceptual Framework of Self-Advocacy in Women with Cancer," *Advances in Nursing Science* 44, no.1 (2021): E1–E13. doi:10.1097/ANS.0000000000000342.

2. Lanlan Zhang et al. "Gender Biases in Estimation of Others' Pain," *Journal of Pain* 22, no. 9 (September 2021). doi 10.1016/j.jpain.2021.03.001.

3. Darcy Banco et al., "Sex and Race Differences in the Evaluation and Treatment of Acute Myocardial Infarction," *Journal of the American Heart Association* 11, no. 10 (May 4, 2022). https://www.ahajournals.org/doi/10.1161/JAHA.121.024199.

4. Nancy N. Maserejian et al., "Disparities in Physicians' Interpretations of Heart Disease Symptoms by Patient Gender: Results of a Video Vignette Factorial Experiment," *Journal of Women's Health* 18, no. 10 (October 2009): 1661–67. https://www.ncbi.nlm.nih.gov/pmc/articles/PMC2825679.

5. Esther H. Chen et al., "Gender Disparity in Analgesic Treatment of Emergency Department Patients with Acute Abdominal Pain," *Academic Emergency Medicine* 15, no. 5 (May 2008): 414–48. https://pubmed.ncbi.nlm.nih.gov/18439195.

6. Paulyne Lee et al. "Racial and Ethnic Disparities in the Management of Acute Pain in US Emergency Departments: Meta-Analysis and Systematic Review," *American Journal of Emergency Medicine* 37, no. 9 (September 2019). https://ajemjournal.com/article/S0735-6757(19)30391-2/fulltext.

7. Kelly M. Hoffman, Sophie Trawalter, Jordan R. Axt, and M. Norman Oliver, "Racial Bias in Pain Assessment and Treatment Recommendations, and

False Beliefs About Biological Differences Between Blacks and Whites,"
Proceedings of the National Academy of Sciences 113, no. 16 (April 19, 2016):
4296–301. https://www.ncbi.nlm.nih.gov/pmc/articles/PMC4843483/.

6: MORE THAN JUST A PRETTY FACE

1. Shelley Emling, "AARP Survey Reveals Disconnect Between Images in Ads and Women's Desire for Realism," AARP, October 22, 2018. https://www.aarp.org/entertainment/style-trends/info-2018/women-beauty-aging-survey.html.
2. David C. Rubin and Dorthe Berntsen, "People over Forty Feel 20% Younger Than Their Age: Subjective Age Across the Lifespan," *Psychonomic Bulletin & Review* 13, no. 5 (October 2006): 776–80. https://www.ncbi.nlm.nih.gov/pmc/articles/PMC3969748/.

7: COMING IN HOT

1. Bisma Tariq et al., "Women's Knowledge and Attitudes to the Menopause: A Comparison of Women over 40 Who Were in the Perimenopause, Post Menopause and Those Not in the Peri or Post Menopause," *BMC Women's Health* 23, no. 1 (August 2023): 460. https://www.ncbi.nlm.nih.gov/pmc/articles/PMC10469514/.
2. Michele Long et al., "Women's Experiences with Provider Communication and Interactions in Health Care Settings: Findings from 2022 KFF Women's Health Survey," KFF (February 22, 2023). https://www.kff.org/womens-health-policy/issue-brief/womens-experiences-with-provider-communication-interactions-health-care-settings-findings-from-2022-kff-womens-health-survey/.
3. Rawan Aljumah, Samantha Phillips, and Joyce C. Harper, "An Online Survey of Postmenopausal Women to Determine Their Attitudes and Knowledge of the Menopause," *Post Reproductive Health* 29, no. 2 (June 2023): 67–84. https://pubmed.ncbi.nlm.nih.gov/36994487/.
4. Jennifer Wolff, "What Doctors Wish Women Knew About Menopause," AARP, July 20, 2018. https://www.aarp.org/health/conditions-treatments/info-2018/menopause-symptoms-doctors-relief-treatment.html.
5. Meryl Davids Landau, "Menopausal Women Are Often Gaslit by the Medical Profession," *Everyday Health*, August 10, 2023. https://www.everydayhealth.com/menopause/menopausal-women-arent-crazy-theyre-just-often-gaslit.
6. Tariq et al., "Women's Knowledge and Attitudes to the Menopause."
7. Lydia Brown, Valerie Brown, Fiona Judd, and Christina Bryant, "It's Not as Bad as You Think: Menopausal Representations Are More Positive in Postmenopausal Women," *Journal of Psychosomatic Obstetrics and Gynecology* 39, no. 4 (December 2018): 281–88. https://pubmed.ncbi.nlm.nih.gov/28937311/.
8. Devon Sanford, "SJF Market Analysis Outlines Startups Disrupting Menopause Care and Opportunities for Investors," SJF Ventures, June 29, 2023. https://sjfventures.com/sjf-ventures-market-analysis-outlines-startups-disrupting-menopause-care-and-opportunities-for-investors/.
9. Grand View Research, "Menopause Market Size, Share & Trends Analysis Report by Treatment (Dietary Supplements, OTC Pharma Products), by Region (North America, Europe, Latin America), and Segment Forecasts, 2024–

2030." https://www.grandviewresearch.com/industry-analysis/menopause
-market.

10. *Nature* editorial, "Women's Health: End the Disparity in Funding,"May 3,
2023. https://www.nature.com/articles/d41586-023-01472-5.

8: I'LL BE THERE FOR YOU

1. Isabel Goddard, "What Does Friendship Look Like in America?" Pew Research Center, October 12, 2023. https://www.pewresearch.org/short-reads
/2023/10/12/what-does-friendship-look-like-in-america/.

2. Maggie Mertens, "Close Friends Can Help You Live Longer but They Can
Spread Some Bad Habits Too," NPR, November 20, 2023. https://www.npr
.org/sections/health-shots/2023/11/20/1214189630/close-friends-can-help
-you-live-longer-but-they-can-spread-some-bad-habits-too.

9: THEY FLEW THE COOP

1. Christoph Becker, Isadora Kirchmaier, and Stefan T. Trautmann, "Marriage,
Parenthood and Social Network: Subjective Well-Being and Mental Health
in Old Age," *PLOS One* 14, no. 7 (July 2019). https://doi.org/10.1371
/journal.pone.0218704.

2. Netta Weinstein, Thuy-vy Nguyen, and Heather Hansen, "What Time
Alone Offers: Narratives of Solitude from Adolescence to Older Adulthood," *Frontiers in Psychology* 12 (November 2021). https://www.ncbi.nlm
.nih.gov/pmc/articles/PMC8591032/.

10: SEX AND THE MIDDLE-AGED WOMAN

1. Susan L. Brown and I-Fen Lin, "The Graying of Divorce: A Half Century
of Change," *Journals of Gerontology: Series B* 77, no. 9 (September 2022):
1710–20. https://academic.oup.com/psychsocgerontology/article/77/9
/1710/6564346.

2. Eunjin Lee Tracy, Jennifer M. Putney, and Lauren M. Papp, "Empty
Nest Status, Marital Closeness, and Perceived Health: Testing Couples'
Direct and Moderated Associations with an Actor-Partner Interdepen-
dence Model," *Family Journal* (Alexandria, Va.) 30, no. 1 (2022): 30–35.
doi:10.1177/10664807211027287.

3. Kira M. Newman, "How Relationship Satisfaction Changes Across Your
Lifetime," *Greater Good Magazine*, February 9, 2022. https://greatergood
.berkeley.edu/article/item/how_relationship_satisfaction_changes_across
_your_lifetime.

4. North American Menopause Society, "Decreased Desire." https://www
.menopause.org/for-women/sexual-health-menopause-online/sexual
-problems-at-midlife/decreased-desire.

5. Harvard Health Publishing, "For Women, Sexuality Changes with Age but
Doesn't Disappear," *Harvard Health Blog*, February 13, 2014. https://www
.health.harvard.edu/blog/for-women-sexuality-changes-with-age-but-doesnt
-disappear-201402137035.

11: THE PARENT TRAP

1. Claire Cain Miller, "Parents Are Highly Involved in Their Adult Children's
Lives, Studies Show," *New York Times*, February 9, 2024. https://www
.nytimes.com/2024/02/09/upshot/parenting-young-adults-relationships.html.

2. Rachel Minkin, Kim Parker, Juliana Mensce Horowitz, and Carolina Aragão, "Parents, Young Adult Children, and the Transition to Adulthood," Pew Research Center, January 25, 2024. https://www.pewresearch.org/social-trends/2024/01/25/parents-young-adult-children-and-the-transition-to-adulthood/.

12: WHAT COULD HAVE BEEN

1. Michael Hardy, "Research: The Road Not Taken," *Mendoza Business Magazine*, Spring 2021. https://bizmagazine.business.nd.edu/issues/2021/spring-2021/research-the-road-not-taken/.
2. Brianna Richardson, "CNBC|SurveyMonkey Poll: International Women's Day 2022," *Curiosity at Work*, February 21, 2022. https://www.surveymonkey.com/curiosity/cnbc-women-at-work-2022/.

13: MINDING MY OWN BUSINESS

1. Kathleen Elkins, "Here's the Age at Which You'll Earn the Most in Your Career," CNBC, August 17, 2017. https://www.cnbc.com/2017/08/17/when-youll-earn-the-most-in-your-career.html.
2. Amy Diehl, Leanne M. Dzubinski, and Amber L. Stephenson, "Women in Leadership Face Ageism at Every Age," *Harvard Business Review*, June 16, 2023. https://hbr.org/2023/06/women-in-leadership-face-ageism-at-every-age.
3. Monica Torres, "Data Reveals An Infuriating Reason Women over 40 Are Held Back at Work," *HuffPost*, July 11, 2023. https://www.huffpost.com/entry/age-discrimination-women_l_64ac0fe0e4b02fb0e6f9d516.
4. Dominic-Madori Davis, "Startups with All-Women Founding Teams Raised Just $1.4B in H1," *TechCrunch*, July 20, 2023. https://techcrunch.com/2023/07/20/all-women-team-funding-h12023/.
5. U.S. Small Business Administration, "National Women's Small Business Month." https://www.sba.gov/about-sba/organization/observances/national-womens-small-business-month.
6. Pierre Azoulay, Benjamin F. Jones, Daniel Kim, and Javier Miranda, "Research: The Average Age of a Successful Startup Founder Is 45," *Harvard Business Review*, July 11, 2018. https://hbr.org/2018/07/research-the-average-age-of-a-successful-startup-founder-is-45.
7. Sukanlaya Sawang, "Why Middle-Aged Entrepreneurs Are Better Than Young Ones," *The Conversation*, June 27, 2018. https://theconversation.com/why-middle-aged-entrepreneurs-are-better-than-young-ones-96297.
8. Adam Grant, "Women Know Exactly What They're Doing When They Use 'Weak Language'," *New York Times*, July 31, 2023. https://www.nytimes.com/2023/07/31/opinion/women-language-work.html.

ABOUT THE AUTHOR

BROOKE SHIELDS is an actress, author, mother, and wife. She is the author of two previous books, *Down Came the Rain* and *There Was a Little Girl*. She resides with her family in New York City, where she was born.